Exhibiting Madness in Museums

Routledge Research in Museum Studies

1. **Contesting Human Remains in Museum Collections**
   The Crisis of Cultural Authority
   Tiffany Jenkins

2. **Museum Gallery Interpretation and Material Culture**
   Edited by Juliette Fritsch

3. **Representing Enslavement and Abolition on Museums**
   Edited by Laurajane Smith, Geoff Cubitt, Ross Wilson and Kalliopi Fouseki

4. **Exhibiting Madness in Museums**
   Remembering Psychiatry through Collections and Display
   Edited by Catharine Coleborne and Dolly MacKinnon

Exhibiting Madness in Museums

Remembering Psychiatry through Collections and Display

Edited by Catharine Coleborne and Dolly MacKinnon

Routledge
Taylor & Francis Group
NEW YORK LONDON

First published 2011
by Routledge
711 Third Ave, New York, NY 10017

Simultaneously published in the UK
by Routledge
2 Park Square, Milton Park, Abingdon, Oxon OX14 4RN

Routledge is an imprint of the Taylor & Francis Group, an informa business

Typeset in Sabon by IBT Global.

Library of Congress Cataloging-in-Publication Data

Exhibiting madness in museums : remembering psychiatry through collections and display / edited by Catharine Coleborne and Dolly MacKinnon.
p. cm.—(Routledge research in museum studies ; 4)
Includes bibliographical references and index.
1. Psychiatry—Museums. 2. Psychiatry—History—Sources. 3. Mental illness—Museums. 4. Mental illness—History—Sources. 5. Psychiatric hospitals—History—Sources. 6. Mentally ill—History—Sources. 7. Museums—Collection management. 8. Museum exhibits. 9. Material culture. I. Coleborne, Catharine. II. MacKinnon, Dolly.
RC454.4.E924 2011
616.89—dc22
2011004439

ISBN: [978-0-415-88092-3] (hbk)
ISBN: [978-0-203-80710-1] (ebk)

Contents

Figures

Figures

Acknowledgements

This book marks a period of sustained intellectual engagement, for both of the editors, with the intersections between the histories of psychiatry and the scholarship around museums and display. We acknowledge and welcome the support and interest of our publishers—Routledge/Taylor & Francis Group—who have fostered this new, interdisciplinary work, as well as injecting ideas into its framework at critical points, including through the discussion of readers' reports. We specifically thank Laura Stearns, our Commissioning Editor, and Stacy Noto, our Editorial Assistant, who have both guided the project through to its completion. Work such as this also depends on the contributions of our ten authors who have stayed with us through the long process of the inception of the project through to the delivery of the manuscript, and have produced fascinating pieces of scholarship and evidence of museum praxis in their individual chapters. As editors and authors, we each visited collections, museums, exhibitions and displays and relied on access to these, and we acknowledge all of the collectors, societies, organisations and institutions who enabled these pieces of research over time. We offer particular thanks below.

As researchers, we have also both worked alongside supportive and interested colleagues over the duration of this project. At the University of Waikato, initially Dr Bronwyn Labrum and later Professor Giselle Byrnes each stimulated Cathy's interest in museums and collections by inviting her to speak to this project in their graduate level paper on public histories. Bronwyn has been an especially interested and keen supporter of this type of research and Cathy has appreciated her contributions and insights. In 2009, Michael Healy produced an excellent Honours dissertation about mental health museums and the World Wide Web which also provoked thinking and discussion in the supervision team around the questions of ethics, display and access to mental health histories. Professor Mark Finnane invited us to speak at a seminar hosted by the Museum of Brisbane and the Centre for Public Culture and Ideas at Griffith University in 2007, which coincided with the 'Remembering Goodna' exhibition discussed in this volume by Jo Besley and Mark himself. Although we spoke about different aspects of these histories, now published as articles in *Health and History* as a Special Issue 'Australian Asylums and their Histories' (11:1, 2009), this event spurred our thinking about this particular publishing project. We thank the participants and audience members who engaged us there in useful discussions about material culture and psychiatric histories.

Over the past few years, Dr Doris Kordes has been a wonderful support to us through communications about mental health and the Kenmore Museum at Goulburn in New South Wales, Australia. Early portions of Cathy's research also benefited from research assistance offered by graduate students in History, including Fiona Kean, and funded by separate contestable research grants from the Faculty of Arts and Social Sciences at the University of Waikato from 2001. It is a pleasure to work with Dolly MacKinnon on our joint ventures and this project has been no exception.

The gestation time and intellectual development for Dolly's research has spanned arts and music faculties at three universities since 1998. Dolly is extremely grateful to her colleagues, especially Professor Elizabeth Malcolm, Dr Lee-Ann Monk, Dr Ann Westmore, Dr Dianne Hall at The University of Melbourne (2002–2010), and also colleagues and students at The Queensland University of Technology (1998–2002) and The University of Queensland (1995–1998). She would also like to thank a number of key people in archives and museums, including Jo Besley at the Museum of Brisbane, Dr Nurin Veis at Museum Victoria, and Laura Brouard at the Lothian Health Services Archive, University of Edinburgh, for their great insights, humour and conversations regarding these collections and exhibitions. Part of Dolly's research for this project has also been supported by two Australian Research Council collaborative research grants (a Discovery grant with Professor Malcolm, and a Linkage grant with Professor Malcolm and Dr Veis), and also a Career Enhancement Fellowship (2008–2010) from The University of Melbourne. Collaborative ventures take research into new, exciting and unchartered waters, and as a testament to this Dolly would like to thank Cathy once again for being such an excellent collaborator on this book, their third co-editing project.

We acknowledge our families: Craig Hight and Cassidy, and Ray Osborne and Alex, for their wonderful support and generosity with their time. Finally, this book would never have been completed without the superb editorial assistance supplied by Dr. Fiona Martin. Fiona's cheerful, tireless and careful work to produce the manuscript to publication stage has made our lives so much easier at crucial stages, and we wish to thank Fiona sincerely for her intellectual and practical contributions to this book.

Catharine Coleborne—*University of Waikato*
Dolly MacKinnon—*University of Queensland*

Part I

Ways of Seeing and Remembering Psychiatry in the Museum

1 Seeing and Not Seeing Psychiatry

Dolly MacKinnon and Catharine Coleborne

How is past psychiatry both seen and obscured? In this volume, we contend that psychiatric practices, as well as those who have been made subject to its regimes, become more visible when we consider both the material and visual cultures produced through and by psychiatric institutions, and also the later representations of these as they are embodied in museums, collections and displays. The more elusive fragments from the world of mental health constitute the basis of this series of individual investigations into past psychiatry. We argue here that the themes of material culture, museums and public display intersect with the dominant scholarship in current histories of psychiatry in new and productive ways. Histories of psychiatry have, broadly speaking, drawn heavily upon textual materials such as the extensive archival remains of institutional medical cultures of the nineteenth century in the form of patient clinical case notes. This collection departs from that tradition and instead takes objects as its central focus. In this way, our collective endeavour is to make visible and audible different views of past psychiatry.

While much has been written on the history of psychiatry, remarkably little has been written about psychiatric collections and their display. The existing literature has either catalogued relevant medical collections, or tended to concentrate on the relatively small number of individual psychiatric art collections worldwide. No study has examined the far more numerous and extensive practices of psychiatric collections, or the material histories of the many individuals, both patients and staff, who lived and worked in these institutions, were incarcerated in them, and whose bodies were made subject to the medical objects that survive in psychiatric collections.

Furthermore, the rise in family history and genealogy research, evidenced by the popularity of television programs such as the Australian, American and British versions of 'Who Do You Think You Are?', has meant that many families have discovered for the first time the institutionalised experiences of family members about whom they previously knew very little. Such individuals have often been left out of the family narrative because only sketchy details are known about their experience, and because mental illness has been stigmatised over time. Hidden from public and private view, these individuals nevertheless lived inside institutions and touched the solid worlds of institutional spaces and material objects.

This collection offers a comparative history of independent and official institutional collections of psychiatric objects in Australia, New Zealand, Canada and the United Kingdom. The leading scholars in this volume investigate the histories of collectors, collections, their display and the reactions to exhibitions of the history of insanity. Linked to the study of medical museums, this work for the first time broadens the study of the history of psychiatry by assessing the significance and importance of the role of twentieth-century psychiatric communities in the preservation, interpretation and representation of the history of mental health through the practices of collecting. Interpreting the purpose and meanings of the psychiatric collection and its display involves engaging with a range of concepts and practices including memory, collections and exhibiting.

Therefore this project draws upon several different explanatory frameworks. In separate essays, authors investigate theories about collecting and collectors; medical museums and psychiatric collections; visual cultures of insanity; photography and institutions; the ethics of exhibiting psychiatric materials; material culture through institutional clothing; the soundscapes of recreation and forms of technology; and through exhibitions of psychiatric institutions, heritage and memories; as well as the collection and exhibition of bodies and body parts on display.

Psychiatric collections play a significant role in histories of twentieth-century psychiatry. These link us to ways of remembering and memorialising psychiatry and experiences of mental illness. Echoing the words of Paul Antze and Michael Lambek, museum scholar Susan M. Pearce writes that '[c]ollections are essentially a narrative of experience'.[1] In these psychiatric collections and their display, we can detect the many possible narratives of the psychiatric experience, and show how these constitute new representations of psychiatric history. Yet some narratives are necessarily more strident than others in these representations. Collecting psychiatry has largely been a private practice conducted within the confines of the institution, and away from the public gaze. Some collections are housed in former psychiatric hospitals, and some are now available online; for instance, the Lost Cases, Recovered Lives exhibition, about found suitcases of psychiatric patients at Willard Hospital for the Insane in New York.[2]

In the second half of the twentieth century, the widespread closures of psychiatric institutions brought specific challenges for psychiatric communities and also broke down the clear distinctions between notions of 'inside' and 'outside' institutional communities.[3] Memories of asylums as concrete places are now all around us. They are especially evident in the recent history-making around psychiatry by former institutional communities. As Antze and Lambek assert, memories 'are never simply records of the past, but are interpretative reconstructions that bear the imprint of local narrative conventions, cultural assumptions . . . and practices.'[4]

Writing about the twentieth-century history of Severalls Hospital in Essex (UK), Diana Gittins notes that to 'try and account for the history of the hospital . . . demands consideration of both space and time, and the interstices and intersections between them.'[5] Cultural and historical geographers have been attuned to these ideas about space and material worlds, and have written about 'post-asylum geographies' in the context of writing about health and place.[6] For example, Alun Joseph, Robin Kearns and Graham Moon argue for 'an expansion of the cultural-geographic interest in the place of memory in the built environment to include abandoned sites of psychiatric treatment'.[7] This scholarship is important for historians of material culture and collecting to consider. Yet although these scholars have demonstrated interest in the spaces of the institution, as well as in mapping the social spaces constructed through psychiatric illness, with some exceptions they have yet to turn their attention to the relationship between psychiatric space, objects and memory or memorialisation.[8]

This particular relationship is at the heart of our discussion about remembering the past of psychiatry, its spaces and their meanings, through its material culture, both visual and auditory. The space of the psychiatric hospital was organised around gendered power relationships. Identities for staff and patients formed within institutional spaces were also constructed through power relations. Objects formed part of this institutional dynamic. Some objects and material culture were handled exclusively by staff. Other objects were reserved for the use of patients: men as well as women, adults and children. Some items were used to treat and/or discipline patients, while others were made by patients and/or staff for either individual or collective use within the asylum. Asylums and later mental hospitals also branded institutional goods to promote the authority of the medical institution and to prevent thefts and pilfering by staff and opportunists.

In writing about the history of collections of psychiatry it is important to recognise that there are two violently opposed schools of thought: those that wish to preserve a form of history, and those who would be happy to see no trace left of the former psychiatric regimes, the buildings and landscape that housed them, as well as any artefacts that relate to these practices. As Peter Beresford observes for Britain '[f]or some survivors, the idea of retaining the bricks and mortar of even one psychiatric hospital may be too painful and they [survivors] want them all razed to the ground.'[9] Thus those that actively collect items for psychiatric collections are consciously choosing to remember and preserve part of their past for posterity. Psychiatric collections, while they comprise evidence of past practices, are really therefore as much about constructing the present and the future of psychiatry. They represent some past actors, but through processes of selection, omission, and oversight, they also obfuscate and obliterate the voices of the majority.

In remembering the asylum and its different communities in the twentieth century, individuals who lived and worked inside an institution have struggled to preserve the physical character of their world. The essays included here consider the way that collections of objects from former psychiatric institutions can play different roles in the construction of psychiatry's histories. They further historicise the very act of collecting and interrogate its meanings across both time and space, with individual chapter contributors from several countries.

Yet, as Nurin Veis suggests in her chapter, the ethical display of psychiatric objects is fraught, as many of the custodians of these collections are all too aware. While many items in these collections are of a medical therapeutic nature, there are also items from everyday life, and in some instances, even personal effects from former patients. Personal property in particular presents the problem of how informed consent for display can be obtained when the patient is either dead or unidentified. These issues, as well as the ongoing housing and maintenance of these objects, continue to plague curators in charge of these significant historic collections. Accessible only by appointment, most of these psychiatric collections are not open to the public, which begs the question, who is the intended audience for these collections? Equally problematic are the reasons that these collections were created and kept. Most recently, mental health users/survivors have questioned the appropriation of their past by the medical and state bodies, as well as individuals, in the creation, collection and constructions of psychiatric history. For many mental health users/survivors the only alternative is to construct, as Beresford advocates, 'a survivor-controlled museum of madness and the psychiatric system.'[10]

Particularly in the twentieth century, as deinstitutionalisation saw the demise of large psychiatric services in favour of community care options and acute hospital ward services, the many diverse and often obsolete records and material culture objects of this trade were kept from the public gaze. Whatever the rationale for the creation of each collection—whether curious and *ad hoc* remnants retained in a store room, active accumulation tracing therapeutic practices over time by staff, or desperate last minute collections of items abandoned in buildings scheduled for demolition—these collections remain controversial. The unifying quality of these collections has been their use in writing the evolutionary history of psychiatry, where the past represents a 'horror' that contrasts with the more enlightened practices of the present. For these reasons, this volume offers the fields of museum studies and the cultural history of mental health a much needed critical study of the many forms and functions of collecting psychiatry, and the place of memory and museums in the constructions of complex histories about psychiatry in the twentieth and twenty-first centuries.

This collection also fills a significant gap and offers a timely analysis of the literature about the history of museums and psychiatric collections, at a time when an increasing number of these psychiatric collections are being made available to the general viewing public for the first time, either in museum exhibitions or via online interpretations. The contributions offered within the covers of this volume aim to provide a contextual account for professionals—including museum curators, historians of psychiatry, medicine and cultural history—as well as the general public, about the ethical responsibilities and benefits of displaying patients' experiences and psychiatry's history in an informed and inclusive way. This timely volume opens a series of debates, which, through the various trajectories discussed within its contents, are intended to guide and inspire those involved in this rapidly growing research field towards innovative new directions in the display of psychiatric collections in the twenty-first century.

Ethical collecting and display are now fundamental considerations of museum acquisition and exhibitions, although this has not always the case. Recent significant global media coverage has been given to the contentious issue of indigenous bodies as subjects of display, along with the presence of cultural artefacts in public and university museums in Britain and Europe. As Shannon Faulkhead and Jim Berg discuss in the context of Victoria, Australia, 'during and after colonial-invasion [*sic*], Koorie graves and cemeteries were desecrated in the name of curiosity, science and research,' and 'Ancestors were removed from their land where they had been placed with care and ceremony, to be housed in metal boxes and cabinets as specimens.'[11] As the Creativespirits website poignantly articulates,

> Imagine you cannot visit the grave of, and pay respect to, members of your family because their remains are not in a cemetery but tucked away in the laboratory of an overseas university, thousands of miles away. Aboriginal remains were removed from graves and burial sites, as well as from hospitals, asylums and prisons throughout the nineteenth century until the late 1940s.[12]

Some early examples of significant and ultimately successful requests for the repatriation of Aboriginal remains within Australia included the cases of Truganini's remains (1976), the Crowther Collections (1985), and other Tasmanian remains (1988) from the Tasmanian Museum and Art Gallery and the return of the Murray Black Collection from The University of Melbourne, Department of Anthropology in the 1980s.[13] The formal cultural recognition of the need for both the repatriation of ancestral bodies and cultural artefacts has now been established in law and is administered by federal and state government bodies, and includes regulating the responsibilities of government museums in both Australia and the United States.[14] Aboriginal, Traditional Owners, Māori and First Nations peoples have had to agitate and petition governments for decades for the return of their ancestors and ancestral belongings. This is especially problematic where artefacts are held in overseas collections.

These events and the practice of collecting highlights a centuries-old culture of the global trafficking in bodies and objects, including those obtained from psychiatric institutions, for public and private museum collections, and the denial of the rights of the very subjects of those collections to have any voice regarding issues of ethical collecting and informed consent. While Aboriginal, Traditional Owners, Māori, and First Nations peoples have pursued their respective fights for the recognition, respect and repatriation of their artefacts and their ancestors' bodies held by institutions around the globe, the vast numbers of patients of former psychiatric institutions represent other voices who have until recently remained silenced regarding the collections created from the remnants of their institutional lives. This is because the construction of a patient's individual identity is far more complex and diverse than the medical label of 'mental illness' implies or allows. Patients are collectively grouped as the mentally ill by health authorities around the world. The facilities inhabited by those suffering from mental illness—where the medical, domestic, work and everyday objects and furnishings of institutional life were in use—have always been the subject of collecting. In the aftermath of deinstitutionalisation, these buildings have now become the *ad hoc* homes for those collections of the material culture remnants of madness.

While many everyday life commodities from the recent and distant past have become the focus of interactive and experiential museum exhibits that meet the burgeoning market of consumable cultural heritage, it comes as no surprise that psychiatry has not been a major contributor to, nor a draw card for, visitors in this field of curating and display. This is primarily for two reasons: the first of which is that very few psychiatric collections are held by public museums and are on permanent display. Catharine Coleborne's chapter shows that many psychiatric collections are held by private, often voluntary and cash-strapped groups that are linked to either a specific institution or to former staff members. Furthermore, these collections are not always open to the general public to browse. The artefacts of psychiatry remain as inaccessible to the broader community now, as they once were when they were in use within psychiatric institutions.

Many psychiatric museums created by medical and general staff around the world are closed to the public. The limited number of psychiatric collections that have been open to the public have met a number of standard responses: large percentages of the viewing public decide to stay away from exhibitions that focus exclusively on mental health history; a voyeuristic proportion of the public simply want to gaze at the mad; and finally, former patients, family members, friends and staff, as well as some members of the general public, are interested in attempting to gain a clearer understanding of the experience of patients and practitioners in psychiatric institutions. Sensitive and compassionate exhibitions about specific institutions have found critical acclaim from sections of the viewing public, including the Remembering Goodna exhibition at Museum of Brisbane in Queensland, Australia, the subject of the chapter by Joanna Besley and Mark Finnane in this volume. However, these successes have been complicated and far outweighed by the large proportion of the general public who voraciously consume the private, fee-entry, worldwide travelling collections, such as Gunter von Hagens' plastination body part shows, as well as his live autopsy shows, some of which have made use of former psychiatric patients' bodies.

As the ways in which the history of psychiatry can be displayed increases through new technological advancements, never before has such a book about the perils and purposes of psychiatric display been so necessary and so apt. This chapter briefly addresses three major over-arching themes in this collection: Ways of Seeing and Remembering Psychiatry in the Museum; Material Culture and Memories of Madness; and Bodies and Fragments. We argue that our use of these themes, and each individual author's intellectual engagement with them, provides a way to address some of the most pressing issues of our time regarding the exhibition and interpretation of the personal experiences of mental illness in the post-institutional age.

WAYS OF SEEING AND REMEMBERING PSYCHIATRY IN THE MUSEUM

Collecting has been a driving force at the centre of the multiple functions of psychiatric institutions over their entire history. Psychiatric institutions around the world shared a common purpose through the changing processes of collecting, purportedly for the benefit of both the community and the individual, either voluntary or involuntary patients in the name of medical science and advances in treatment into institutional systems. Coleborne's chapter suggests that close investigations of separate psychiatric collections can reveal much about their meanings for collectors, exhibition curators and audiences in museums. It is through collections and their multiple interpretations that we might find out more about the material cultures and histories of institutional worlds and lives. The very 're-membering' of 'things' can tell us about the absences in historical scholarship in a field that is so focused on textual representations it has ignored the physical worlds and memories of the insane.[15] Collectors and their motivations, too, need to be understood in their historical context, but also as part of an ongoing series of dilemmas about the politics of representing the histories of those confined as insane.

As Barbara Brookes shows in her chapter asylums were quick to make use of new technologies and, in the case of photography, patients were photographed in order to demonstrate the typology of madness. Pathology examples were also photographed and circulated among medical staff within and across institutions in the interests of scientific advancement. Over time, however, the function of photography of the asylum inhabitants shifted. In the twenty-first century, the individual patient portraits that were understood to be collective representations of forms of madness now represent an individual face for one of the millions of patients who passed through or died in these institutions across the British Empire and beyond. Brookes also powerfully evokes another reading of the presence and absence of patient subjectivities through her discussion of contemporary photographic exhibitions of former and now often derelict psychiatric facilities.

Brookes' chapter also reminds us that the need for an ethical framework for exhibiting psychiatric materials lies at the centre of any visual display of the material culture of psychiatry's past. Within the context of ethically displaying psychiatric objects, museum curator Nurin Veis discusses the design and establishment of a framework for ethical practice regarding highly sensitive exhibits in a piece which has broad application across museology.

MATERIAL CULTURE AND MEMORIES OF MADNESS

We have been arguing that highlighting the past and current uses of material culture tells us more about the way insanity and its institutions have been remembered. A significant proportion of this book focuses on the various kinds of material objects and cultural remains of institutional life. We evoke here debates about the 'material turn' in historical and cultural studies scholarship which partly calls for historians in particular to recognise the powerful presence of objects in everyday life, and their relationships to regimes of power, as well as their meanings for historical research and writing.[16] It is not only museums that provide an interpretive context, then, for thinking about objects.[17] Historians might also, like their curator colleagues, think about the ways that objects tell stories and offer up new narratives of past worlds. Bronwyn Labrum's chapter 'materialises' clothing from psychiatric institutions and shows how additional views and aspects of their histories can shed new light on older narratives of mental health. For Labrum, clothing allows us to 'see' beyond histories of the asylum as built environments, and move inside the domestic worlds and lives of patients and staff alike, providing 'new materialisations of power and subjectivity' in the process. Labrum also demonstrates that although the material culture of each psychiatric collection is unique, each captures aspects of the gendered landscape of the institution.

Like Labrum, Dolly MacKinnon reminds us that the material culture in use in these institutions was not only visual. For MacKinnon, it could also be part of the auditory world of the asylum. Used in specific and gender-select ways, sound objects—that is pianos, gramophone records and radios that generated music and relayed broadcasts inside the asylum—formed part of the regulated, gendered soundscape of the institution. Sporting carnivals, including cricket and curling, contributed to the soundscape of recreation within the asylum grounds. Musical objects, sporting equipment, and the sanctioned material culture of religious worship in Australian and Scottish asylums were understood by the medical authorities to constitute different forms of recreation. These practices, however, are unevenly represented in collections, with some forms of recreation leaving no material culture traces at all.

Furthermore, museum display practices use either individual auditory commentary guides, or general gallery soundscapes to accompany specialist or general exhibitions respectively. For psychiatric collections, MacKinnon contends that, where possible, the inclusion of re-activated sound objects can contextualise individual and collective patient experiences in more meaningful ways. MacKinnon articulates, just as Labrum suggests, that these silenced, under-utilised objects within closed museum displays have much more to tell us about the segregated gendered landscape of the asylum from the mid-nineteenth to the mid-twentieth century.

Psychiatric hospitals have also become new sites for the memorialisation of the past treatments and experiences of the insane. In their chapter, Nathan Flis and David Wright show how a wider, global project to memorialise past psychiatry can be witnessed through the shifting sites of memory embodied in the commemoration and preservation of institutional spaces and physical landmarks. Taking Canadian cultural memory projects around mental health as their starting point, they examine different forms of memory and madness in both scholarly and activist contexts. By relating the field of memory studies to the questions we raise in this collection, Flis and Wright offer examples of material memories that threaten to expose stereotypical renditions of psychiatric history, also playing with the scholarly trope of 'museums of madness'.[18] They too show that 'asylum museums' are no longer the dominant mode for a discovery of the material cultures of mental health.

Although the 'asylum museum' might now be an outmoded concept, other authors provide evidence of the role of the carefully conceptualised museum exhibition. In their chapter Joanna Besley and Mark Finnane examine the 'generative potential' of exhibitions which take mental health as their subject. The Museum of Brisbane exhibition in Queensland, Australia, opened up the institutional world of psychiatry to scrutiny to a broad public audience and involved extensive research surrounding the history of the former psychiatric institution first known as Goodna, and later referred to as Woolston Park Hospital. This place was the largest institution for the confinement of the insane from the nineteenth century and its lingering presence in Queensland memory makes it a significant and compelling example of the potential in exhibiting 'madness'. In their detailed reading of their own exhibition, Besley, a museum curator and Finnane, an academic historian noted in the international field of histories of mental health, reflect on the powerful meanings of this memory work for participants, visitors, researchers and past clients of institutions. The many vivid visitor responses to the exhibition attest to the importance of remembering the material spaces of institutional life, as well as their histories for individuals who had only a passing relationship to the site and its meanings over time. We argue that this process is critical to gaining better understandings of psychiatric treatment.

BODIES AND FRAGMENTS

Once inside the institutional system, over time, the scrutiny of patients' bodies generated further collections of medical data in the forms of text, photographic evidence, and even bodies and body parts. Two chapters illustrate these issues well: Helen MacDonald and D. Gareth Jones offer arguments about the bodies of the insane becoming museum artefacts. Once dead, patients' bodies were usually displayed, without their or their families' knowledge or consent, for the amassing of large medical collections of skeletal and pathology samples, taken through the process of post mortems, dissection, and medical discovery. These authors demonstrate for Australia, Germany and New Zealand the disturbing ease with which this either clandestine, or publicly sanctioned, collecting was achieved, and the most disturbing way in which the law at various times enabled such practices to thrive in the nineteenth and twentieth centuries.

Furthermore, as MacDonald's body of work skillfully demonstrates, these skeletal and pathology samples were part of a global network of personal and institutional collecting. When psychiatric institutions faced amalgamation and/or closure, another process of retrospective preservation of the material culture (including skeletal remains and pathology samples) of the histories of professional groups and work practices generated a new form of institutional collecting.

Our volume ends with a chapter about new ways of seeing the lived experiences of mental illness inside a psychiatric secure unit. Fiona R. Parrott's chapter provides a rich ethnographic account of the ways in which psychiatric patients in the contemporary era have made use of 'things' and material objects in their everyday lives. A significant absence that the process of collecting the material culture of psychiatry has largely failed to redress is that of the individual patient experience. Therefore Parrott's chapter, with its intimate and personal accounts offered by patients about their environment is a fitting point both to end with, and also launch off from. It returns our focus to Beresford's advocacy for 'a survivor-controlled museum of madness and the psychiatric system.'[19] Parrott's work, along with the other contributions within this volume, is a testament to the new directions that psychiatric collecting and the retrospective displays of psychiatry's past must take if it is to be truly representative of the vast majority of those women, children, and men it ultimately should seek to represent.

NOTES

1. Susan M. Pearce, *Collecting in Contemporary Practice* (London: Sage, 1998), 412.
2. See: http://www.mentalhealthstigma.com/documentaries.html, and the book about this collection by Darby Penney and Peter Stastny, 2008 accessed April 1, 2011.
3. Diana Gittins, *Madness in its Place: Narratives of Severalls Hospital, 1913–1997* (London: Routledge, 1998), 57.

4. Paul Antze and Michael Lambek, eds., *Tense Past: Cultural Essays in Trauma and Memory* (London: Routledge, 1996), vii.
5. Gittins, *Madness in its Place*, 5.
6. Hester Parr and Chris Philo, *'A Forbidding Fortress of Locks, Bars and Padded Cells': The Locational History of Mental Health Care in Nottingham*, Historical Geography Research Series 32 (London: Historical Geography Research Series, 1996) 1–98; Hester Parr and Chris Philo, "Mapping 'Mad' Identities," in *Mapping the Subject: Geographies of Cultural Transformation*, ed. Steve Pile and Nigel Thrift, (London: Routledge, 1996), 199–225; Hester Parr, "Bodies and Psychiatric Medicine: Interpreting Different Geographies of Mental Health," in *Mind and Body Spaces: Geographies of Illness, Impairment and Disability*, ed. Ruth Butler and Hester Parr (London: Routledge, 1999), 181–202. See also a Special Issue of *Health and Place* on this topic: 6.3 (2000).
7. Alun E. Joseph, Robin A. Kearns, and Graham Moon, "Recycling Former Psychiatric Hospitals in New Zealand: Echoes of Deinstitutionalisation and Restructuring," *Health & Place* 15 (2009): 86.
8. See for instance Robin Kearns, Alun E. Joseph and Graham Moon, "Memorialisation and Remembrance: On Strategic Forgetting and the Metamorphosis of Psychiatric Asylums into Sites for Tertiary Educational Provision," *Social and Cultural Geography* 11, no. 8 (2010): 731–749.
9. National Empowerment Center—Articles, "Peter Beresford on the Need for a Survivor-Controlled Museum of Madness", 2008, http://www.power2u.org/articles/history-project/museum.html accessed April 1, 2011.
10. "Peter Beresford on the Need for a Survivor-Controlled Museum of Madness," 2008, http://www.power2u.org/articles/history-project/museum.html accessed April 1, 2011.
11. Shannon Faulkhead and Jim Berg, with Lynette Russell, Ross L. Jones and Jason Eades, *Power and the Passion: Our Ancestors Return Home* (Melbourne, Victoria: Koorie Heritage Trust, 2010), xi.
12. "Aboriginal Remains Repatriation," http://www.creativespirits.info/aboriginalculture/ people/aboriginal-remains.html (accessed November 18, 2010).
13. European Network for Indigenous Australian Rights (ENIAR), "Repatriation of Aboriginal Human Remains," http://www.eniar.org/ repatriation.html (accessed November 18, 2010).
14. For the Federal Government in Australia see M. Truscott, "Repatriation of Indigenous Cultural Property," paper prepared for the 2006 Australian State of the Environment Committee, Department of Environment and Heritage, Canberra, http://www.environment.gov.au/soe/2006/publications/emerging/repatriation/index.html (accessed November 18, 2010); for the Federal Government in the United States see *The Native American Graves Protection and Repatriation Act* (NAGPRA), 1990, http://www.nps.gov/nagpra/ (accessed November 18, 2010).
15. See Bjørnar Olsen, "Material Culture after Text: Re-Membering Things," *Norwegian Archaeological Review* 36, no.2 (2003): 87–104.
16. The term is also used to refer to the turn to thinking about the material effects of power and the rediscovery of historical materialism. See *Material Powers: Cultural Studies, History and the Material Turn*, ed. Tony Bennett and Patrick Joyce (London: Routledge, 2010).
17. Robert Berkhofer, *Fashioning History: Current Practices and Principles* (New York: Palgrave Macmillan, 2008), 142.
18. See Andrew Scull, *Museums of Madness: The Social Organization of Insanity in Nineteenth-Century England* (London: Allen Lane, 1979).
19. "Peter Beresford on the Need for a Survivor-Controlled Museum of Madness," 2008, http://www.power2u.org/articles/history-project/museum.html accessed April 1, 2011.

2 Collecting Psychiatry's Past
Collectors and Their Collections of Psychiatric Objects in Western Histories

Catharine Coleborne

INTRODUCTION

Psychiatric patients confined in hospitals for the insane in the nineteenth century ate 'cold greasy food' from simple bowls, served from a tin container.[1] They wore shapeless clothing of blue and white galatea, and when they were able to adorn it with more decoration, for formal occasions, they did so.[2] Some patients who exhibited violent or harmful behaviours were restrained by camisoles or straitjackets, and others were cuffed using strong, leather wrist or ankle shackles. Inmates who were placed in seclusion were also reputedly very strong and often scratched words and symbols into the painted walls of their cells. Words written about these inmates were entered into large, leather-bound folios by attendants and medical staff. Much of this physical evidence of the lives of psychiatric patients survives in collections of material culture—collections of 'stuff' from the lived worlds of the confined—which contain objects from the late nineteenth century into the middle of the twentieth century. There are many such collections of objects around the world; they retain a haunting significance to all those touched by the histories of mental illness, and provide lingering reminders of the sometimes frightening histories of mental hospitals, treatments and abuses of hospital inmates, and the dull daily routines of institutional life. This chapter considers these material remnants of past psychiatry through a close examination of three specific collections, but with reference to wider, ongoing practices of psychiatric collecting and display.

One of the most powerful indicators of the relevance of history to public audiences is the continuing engagement with museum spaces for new social histories.[3] Academic historians have already learned much from the way that histories and material culture are now displayed to visitors, who both observe and contribute to history making in museum settings.[4] Museums and their social history curators have trained their gaze on instructive, themed exhibitions for a broad audience base. Exhibitions of mental health histories are among the themes presented to public audiences, with museum curators reasserting the traditional educative function of the museum exhibition in such displays, as well as engaging with the sometimes-fraught politics around mental health histories.[5] Museums, therefore, traditionally homes for collections of objects, have found innovative ways to showcase their often curious collections through exhibitions to public audiences, such as combining online displays with physical exhibits.[6] But collections, too, have lives of their own. They are not always displayed, but are sometimes doomed to a private and silent existence in the basements of large museums, or other small spaces. This chapter focuses on collections of psychiatric objects, the impetus behind them, as well as their meanings and significance as collections. It draws upon specific examples from several collections in Australia and New Zealand, also touching on aspects of their display and the public reception to exhibitions of mental health history, but also places these in an international context of medical museums and collections.[7] By utilising museum scholars' understandings of 'making history', as well as exploring the scholarly impact of the 'material turn', this chapter examines the often obscured function of the psychiatric collection in historical context.[8]

Here, I propose a new strand in the literature about the history of collecting and collectors, and argue for a theory of this type of collecting that makes sense of the need to preserve the past of psychiatry. I explore some of the ways we might begin to understand these collectors and their collections to bring some clarity to their purpose and their meanings. Collecting has received specific attention in the field of museum studies, and has been the subject of a range of interesting studies. Collecting was historically associated with the Western appropriation of the 'exotic other', with early collectors ranging from imperialist explorers and voyagers to scientific men in the eighteenth century, with a professionalisation of collecting practices in the nineteenth century through the institution of the museum. The focus was on ethnographic exhibits: museum exhibitions were epitomised by the large collections of, for example, the famous Pitt Rivers Museum at Oxford which houses objects from colonised peoples all over the world. What historians aptly describe as Renaissance to modern practices of 'collecting the world' became defining activities for nation states by the nineteenth century.[9] Similarly, Henrietta Riegel argues that such exhibitions inscribed both a 'politics of difference' and a specific mode of 'viewing' inside the space of the museum, defining a new 'power relation' in the process.[10]

More recently, the scholarly turn to understanding the collections of the mundane, the ordinary or the objects of 'everyday life' has shaped some of the appreciation of the function of collecting as a practice.[11] Russell W. Belk, for example, explores collecting practices across time in the context of the rise of the consumer society in the Western world, using case-studies of individual collectors in the twentieth century as diverse as collectors of beer cans, tattoos, and postal histories.[12] Susan M. Pearce examines the 'urge to collect', along with writers who explore the psychological desire for objects and things.[13] Their ideas about collecting inform my interpretation of psychiatric collecting, as I will explain.

Psychiatry in the western world was characterised by a dramatic shift in the twentieth century. Large public institutions for the treatment of the mentally ill, some with long cultural and physical histories reaching into the early nineteenth century, were progressively closed or limited to small intakes. These processes of institutional closure caused pain for sectors of the psychiatric community, among them staff and patients, some of whom had experienced the institution as a home. Others felt that the institutional closures were justified and overdue. Either way, the importance of documenting these places and their histories suddenly became critical. Nursing staff were particularly at the forefront of collecting the material culture of their workplace. Some buildings became heritage sites and turned into small museums with former staff lobbying for their survival.[14] Most of this activity was conducted by 'amateur' historians and curators.

This phenomenon of psychiatric collecting in the wake of deinstitutionalisation might be seen as a continuation of the tradition of the medical museum, as I will explore further.[15] However, such collecting also embodies its own meanings, as small collections and some museums have not always been attached to medical teaching hospitals or universities. They remain oddities, mostly poorly resourced and are often peripatetic. Their champions have been older and mostly retired members of the former institutional workplace communities from which they sprang. In addition, few large public museums have successfully displayed this type of material, with some exceptions, as the chapters in this volume by Nurin Veis and Jo Besley and Mark Finnane suggest. Therefore, as I argue, the particular role of psychiatric collections, whether or not such collections are displayed, can tell us more about psychiatric history. Their very existence tells us about the function of memory, the uses of the collection in the production of collective memories, and about the role of objects in the lives of their collectors. I also suggest that by addressing this form of psychiatric collecting, we might add to the existing scholarship about interpreting collecting activities and collections themselves.

PSYCHIATRIC COLLECTIONS AND THE MEDICAL MUSEUM

Considering their ubiquitous presence in teaching hospitals and their lengthy histories, medical museums have received surprisingly little scholarly attention from museum studies scholars. Ken Arnold has carved out the field in his work, arguing that medical displays in museums have the potential to influence audiences because of their tremendous visual power, and have contemporary relevance to the general public of debates about health, medicine, and ethics. In addition, medicine reaches audiences because it touches all of our lives; it is, in fact, intrinsically interesting.[16] In other words, Arnold says, medicine might have a long history of being a privileged knowledge for specialist practitioners, but it also appeals to the viewer in more fundamental ways. Arnold reminds us that there is a lengthy tradition of medicine in the museum. Doctors themselves were curators of exhibits, often cabinets of empirical scientific value in their context. There was a purpose to medical collections: they were used in teaching and to educate practitioners about techniques and substances with healing properties. Particularly by the nineteenth century, when medical societies had begun to professionalise their activities, such collections performed an important role in the creation and maintenance of medical knowledge. This took on specific meanings in the colonial context, where the networks of medical practitioners and institutions were shaped by British and Scottish medical traditions, and where the value of such traditions was arguably expressed through teaching and museological practices.[17]

There were distinct periods in the development of the medical museum, as Arnold also shows. Collections were used by some publically-funded museums to educate people about health and hygiene in the mid-twentieth century. Later in the period, many Western countries have a large number of museums with medical collections, with Arnold noting around 200 in Britain by the mid-1990s. In Australia and New Zealand alone, a Health and Medicine Museums group operated from the 1990s until 2006, and was part of a wider network of museums and professionals.[18] The nature of these medical collections supports Arnold's view that medical collecting became extremely broad and inclusive in the latter half of the twentieth century, reflecting shifts in museum collecting more generally, as well as changing conceptions of what constitutes 'health' with the rise of discourses of public health.

However, like the history of psychiatry itself, which is seen as a sub-theme in the wider field of the history of medicine, collections of psychiatric objects need to be considered in a slightly different context. Although it has been part of the story of public health, the history of mental health has been shaped largely through institutions and institutional histories. With the closure of the majority of institutional spaces for the treatment of mental health, a more dramatic rupture occurred in the historical narrative of psychiatric treatment. While health and medicine continue to change rapidly, hospitals still play a major role in the understanding of medicine and its application. Yet practices of psychiatry are now more diffuse, not located in any one site. This means that the urgency associated with the documentation of its history has in part determined the motivations of its narrators, and in the case of objects, the motivations of the collectors of material culture.

There are parallels, though, between medical collecting and psychiatric collecting, including the broad definition of the materials being collected. These are well illustrated through the example of the Charles Brothers Collection of psychiatric objects. The collection takes its name from the psychiatrist Dr Charles Brothers who practiced in Victoria, Australia, in the mid-twentieth century and who began collecting objects, together with his psychiatrist colleagues, in the 1950s. Brothers himself was part of the push for a modern professional identity for psychiatrists in Australia between the late 1940s and the 1960s. He was instrumental in founding the Australasian Association of Psychiatrists, was President of this organization in 1949, and died in 1963.[19] Brothers, along with Dr Eric Cunningham Dax, who was Chairman of the Mental Health Authority, and Dr Herbert Bauer, Superintendent of Kew Mental Hospital, saw the mental health institutions in the 1950s as places in serious decline. The buildings were dilapidated, neglected, and along with some treatments and practices inside institutions, in need of refurbishment and reform. Elsewhere, I write about the significance of these perceptions and the changing landscape of psychiatry to the formation of the collection that was later known as the Charles Brothers Collection. It was precisely this 'cleaning up' of a range of institutional sites which led to the rescue of objects deemed significant to the men who practiced psychiatry at this time.[20]

The Brothers Collection of over 700 items includes sub-collections of apothecary jars, medical instruments, clothing and patient restraint garments from the nineteenth century. Collecting ranged over all aspects of daily institutional life, as well as medical treatments representing different eras of medicine and psychiatry. The interpretation of the collecting, undertaken by subsequent generations of medical and museum curators, emphasises the material evidence of the physical environment of the institutions in Victoria from the late nineteenth century into the twentieth century period.[21] This collection offers rich potential for exhibition precisely because it includes such a wide range of objects, and yet it has rarely been exhibited.[22]

Like the Brothers Collection, which demonstrates the relationship between psychiatric and medical collections, the Mental Health Museum of Western Australia (MHMWA) is a collection which draws upon more than one institutional site and its material objects. It differs from the Brothers Collection in that its collectors have been retired psychiatric nursing staff who became active as collectors in the period of institutional closures in the late 1990s, with the formal collection opening in 1998. In Western Australia, the major public mental health institution of Graylands Hospital (formerly Claremont Asylum) had begun the process of deinstitutionalisation by reorganising its provision of mental health care into different physical sites, and gradually reducing numbers of inpatient beds. Historical artefacts and documents dating back to the late nineteenth century were found discarded at a local dump, and the salvaging of additional objects began with the concerted attention of a few individuals who were concerned about mental health heritage and its disappearance. This extensive but uncatalogued collection of records, photographs, memorabilia, medical objects and equipment has been housed at Graylands Hospital, and partially exhibited as I describe below. However, despite the fact that its collectors have made efforts to professionalise their collecting practices and their policies, its existence has been marginal and under threat.[23]

In New Zealand, the Porirua Hospital Museum (PHM) houses and displays a collection on site in a former part of the Porirua Hospital, the oldest surviving ward of 'F' Block. The museum collection, founded in 1987, represents the remnants of the practice of psychiatry at the hospital, and like the MHMWA, was begun by former psychiatric nursing staff and is maintained by the Friends of the PHM. Again, the hundreds of objects in this collection range from the late nineteenth century to the twentieth century. Uncatalogued, the objects are on display by appointment, and include farm objects, medical equipment, items reflecting sport, leisure and recreation, case-books, registers, as well as clothing. Significantly, this museum recreates a Seclusion Room for visitors.[24]

These three collections represent shifts in thinking about psychiatry over time, but also in practices of collecting. The collectors range from the psychiatrists who were themselves involved in reforming institutional care, to former nursing staff whose relationships to the sites they worked at were different in that they had little to do with policy or change, but were more connected with daily work practices inside institutions and their interactions with patients. Their shared goal to rescue and maintain psychiatric histories through material objects and their aim to engage with the heritage of institutional sites, marks them out as enthusiastic but 'amateur' collectors of everyday life, with some continuum from the Brothers Collection of the 1950s, but an obvious shift in practices to the 1990s with the self-trained collectors at the MHMWA. As I argue in more detail below, the meanings of these three collections for their collectors, and their various audiences, hold clues to their relevance to psychiatric collections more broadly.

While I focus here only on the three collections described above, there are other collections in Australia and New Zealand. Of these, some share similarities with my three case studies. The Kenmore Hospital Museum at Goulburn in New South Wales, Australia, described in the chapter for this volume by Bronwyn Labrum, operates in a similar way to Porirua, and is also housed in a former hospital ward. Themed exhibitions reach an interested public of locals and tourists. Other 'collections' have been assembled expressly for their use in themed exhibitions. The history of Goodna Mental Hospital was exhibited at Museum of Brisbane, and is explored in this volume in Besley and Finnane's chapter. Kew Asylum Museum in Melbourne, a heritage site, contains records salvaged during building and the redevelopment of the former hospital site in the mid-1990s, and includes archival materials, and a 'historical walk' for visitors.[25] For an exhibition of the Tokanui Mental Hospital (1912–1997), at the Te Awamutu Museum located in New Zealand's North Island, curator Stephanie Lambert used a range of objects gathered from community members, oral histories, photographs, and objects in the museum's own collection, including an Official Visitor's Book.[26]

Research suggests, unsurprisingly, that international psychiatric collections tend to be based on former institutional sites.[27] However, the three Australasian examples I use here stand out as 'collections' with coherent identities and collector histories within the international context, perhaps reflecting the particular meanings of heritage in those places. Indeed, the attention paid to 'heritage' in debates around public histories in Australia and New Zealand reminds us that to understand collecting practices and collections, we also need to engage with public history as a specific sub-discipline, as well as with debates about built heritage.[28] In the remainder of this chapter I turn to the ways we might appreciate and interpret the meanings of these collections and their objects for different users and audiences.

THE MEANINGS OF THE PSYCHIATRIC COLLECTION

So far I have suggested that psychiatric collections occupy a curious relationship to medical collections in that they represent a new era of medical collecting based in the motivations of new collectors. These new collectors have been enthusiastic amateurs in terms of contemporary museology, and yet, unlike collectors from earlier eras, have in some instances worked within available professional frameworks for their collecting, including seeking museum training and advice about the formulation of collecting policies, and engaging with the principles of museum display. While continuities with the medical collection and its historical role do exist—witnessed through the idea that the psychiatric collection might, for instance, perform an educative function for trainee doctors and public audiences alike—psychiatric collections also represent historical rupture and change brought about through the process of institutional closures. But what do these arguably 'odd' collections of mouth gags, wrist and ankle shackles, bowls, jackets, sporting equipment, locks and keys, and medicine bottles mean? What is their purpose?

Objects have been 'documents of reality' for their collectors in this field.[29] Touching, holding and viewing objects from former workplaces—sites being rescued as spaces for the care of the mentally ill following their widespread condemnation—has had a therapeutic value for some of their collectors. For other audiences, including former clients of the psychiatric, such objects symbolize fear, serving as reminders of past experiences of brutal and lonely institutional spaces. The interpretation of psychiatric objects depends upon their curator or collector, as well as their audience. From this point of view, the collections that receive little public exposure risk limited interpretation. Each of the three collections I examine here has been displayed in some form, though rarely. In the following sections I comment on the many different 'meanings' that might be ascribed to these collections before analysing their significance as 'hidden objects' in the world of collecting.

For Collectors

When collectors of psychiatric objects have reflected on their motives, their passion, and their decisions, their views can also tell us more about the meaning of these collections. Pearce defines collecting through a diagram of the relationship between the 'enclosed and private world of the individual' and the process of collecting as one way of 'living with chaos and turning it into sense.'[30] If collecting marks a passage through life, as Pearce suggests, then the group collecting of former psychiatric staff—incorporating the individual aspirations and personal motivations of those in the group—certainly speaks to the wider context of anxieties produced around institutional closure, as I argue elsewhere.[31] Collectors repeatedly indicate their emotional responses to their work. While their efforts to become skilled in museum curatorial practices shows a keenness to professionalise their enthusiasm, as well as a realisation that this might also enhance their success in displaying and storing material objects, collectors have mostly focused on their social responsibilities to their work, the very profound connections to their former workplaces as communities, as well as the possible educational function of their collections. For example, both the MHMWA and the PHM Friends have developed collection policies and undertaken museum and curatorial training in their specific contexts. The collectors of the Charles Brothers Collection had opportunities to reflect on their collecting with the staff at the old Museum of Victoria, with Elizabeth Willis' interviews with individual men such as Eric Cunningham Dax deposited in the archival collection of the Melbourne Museum.[32]

For Museum Exhibition Curators

Within the museum studies field, objects are central to the ways in which museums create and present historical narratives. The three elements of this process are representation, space, and audience.[33] These elements provide a useful framework for understanding aspects of the display of psychiatric collections. Dominant cultural representations of psychiatric institutions have come from films and novels, with the strong tendency for exaggeration of the repressive aspects of institutional life, reinforcing the power relationship implicit in the experience of mental illness.[34] How might mental health treatment be represented differently? The melancholic aspects of institutional life are difficult to avoid. It is no longer possible to present an entirely positive narrative of the institution—if ever one existed—but current museum representations of histories of mental health, via collections, do tend to weave both aspects of these representational practices together. Collections contain both gruesome objects and items which provide more hopeful interpretations of the histories of the institutionalised.

The spaces where such collections are both found and exhibited also matters: professional museums are an interpretive context, but should objects remain in heritage settings where they are most explicable, such as the example of the Porirua Hospital Museum? The Brothers Collection was for some years displayed in a mental health teaching context in the Mental Health Library at Royal Park Hospital in Melbourne. In 1986, this collection was transferred from the Department of Mental Health to the

Museum of Victoria, where it remains, though now subsumed within a larger collection.[35] The audiences for these collections and their display were already aware of mental health policy and practice, suggesting a level of understanding of the objects. However, such an audience might focus on the medical meanings of the collection, rather than its wider implications. An overview of the collection produced in 1986 suggests that it had several gaps, including objects relating to the histories of children, entertainment and occupational therapy, absences which could be explained by the provenance of objects dating predominantly to the 1940s. In addition, this collection emphasizes the custodial orientation of mental hospitals to the early 1950s, and therefore any display of these objects would possibly reproduce older stereotypes of historical understanding.[36]

In her sensitive interpretation of the Brothers Collection overall, former Museum of Victoria curator Elizabeth Willis shows how objects require a multilayered interpretation, placement in a wider historical context, and some imaginative leaps of guesswork. Examples from this collection, such as the female patient's canvas straitjacket that has been mended several times, with someone adding a soft fabric to the collar to prevent neck chafing, evoke emotional responses.[37] Willis also casts a cool eye over the gap between rhetoric and practice in hospitals for the insane over a long period of time when it was well known that institutions were poorly resourced; for her, objects reflect a history of scarcity and deprivation. One particular aspect of the Brothers Collection which also shapes its meanings is the fact that curators identified that the period from 1930 to 1950 is severely under-represented in the collection, highlighting 'the worst phases of care of the mentally ill'.[38] They went as far as to say that 'the exhibits should not be displayed if at all possible as a "chamber of horrors", patients suffered terribly, and the hospitals were dreaded and awful establishments, however a well-balanced, and socially historical perspective should be sought'.[39] By contrast, the PHM collection does exhibit objects and stories from this era, including 1930s insulin treatments and ECT machines from the 1940s.

Objects from the Brothers Collection were also displayed in a small exhibition in the Medical History Museum at the Brownless Biomedical Library at the University of Melbourne in 1998 and 1999. A Closed World: The Asylum System in Victoria 1848 to 1920 was an exhibition constructed around themes including identifying insanity; early institutions in Victoria; changing medical treatments and patient populations; official inquiries; and patient support and advocacy. As curator of this exhibition, my own intention was to showcase historical records and aspects of past psychiatric treatment often overlooked.[40] The title of the exhibition, A Closed World, was my preference, given the propensity of similar displays to use terms such as 'out of mind, out of sight', although the so-called 'closed' nature of this institutional world was also questioned in the exhibition. At that stage, the process of opening up this world included a discussion of the ways, for instance, patients were caught in a web of institutional language and knowledge through official reports and patient casebooks. Exhibiting textual objects and sources was something I understood as a historian, but I also drew upon the expertise of a museum curator to explore for the first time the use of objects to tell stories. By exhibiting objects including clothing, such as restraining garments as well as everyday dress (a pyjama jacket and a warder's suit), patient eating utensils (aluminium bowls and forks),

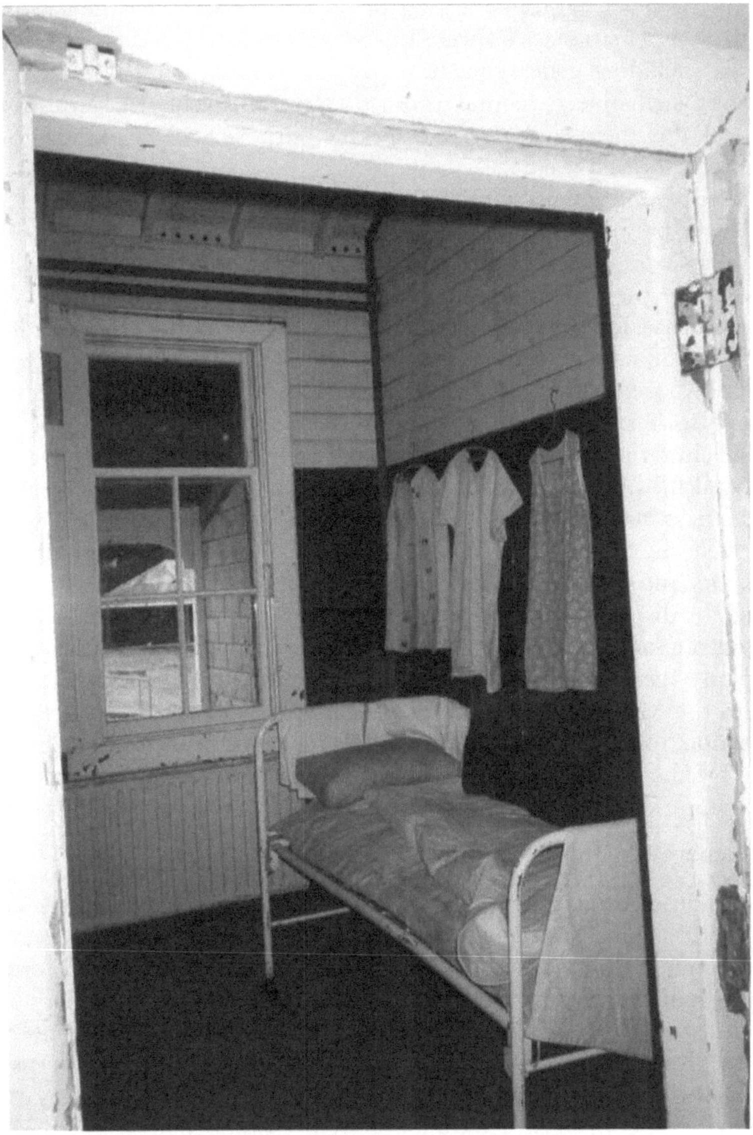

Figure 2.1 Interior room at the Porirua Hospital Museum, New Zealand. *Source*: Author's photograph, 2002.

recreational items (a ball and a tobacco tin) and a letter spike for the superintendent's use, we managed to convey—even fleetingly—an everyday life of institutional confinement in the period.

Medical objects were also displayed and these garnered interest from both medical and non-medical visitors to the exhibition. In many ways these objects were more difficult to weave into the narrative of a social world of insanity and its institutions in colonial Victoria, since they were part of the much larger collection of objects gathered by the 1950s and 1960s by psychiatrists who were interested in medical treatments in institutions, including general medical instruments for non-psychiatric uses. However, such objects remind us of the status of psychiatric institutions as 'medical' and thereby also serve a specific purpose in the Charles Brothers Collection for this reason.

This opening up of 'closed' historical institutional worlds in the late 1990s was paralleled elsewhere. For the Mental Health Museum of WA, a small display of objects at the Claremont Library in Perth in 1998 signalled the work of the collectors to a wider audience. This was followed by an exhibition at Claremont Museum in 1999. Out of Mind—Out of Sight was an exhibition curated by Lillian Hankel for a 'community access gallery'. Like the Closed World exhibition, it also covered the social and political contexts for institutions, this time for the state of Western Australia, reaching back into the colonial era and focusing on treatments for patients. It also displayed medical objects, such as electro-convulsive therapy objects, but placed these in their wider social context.[41] In this case, as with the example described above, the collectors were not in control of the exhibition. The collectors and former psychiatric staff identified with the MHMWA welcomed the display, but also felt disappointed that it did not lead to any permanent site for the collection to be stored or exhibited. By contrast, Porirua Hospital Museum is perhaps fortunate, given the somewhat peripatetic history of the MHMWA, and the comparatively hidden history of Brothers Collection, to be located on site and open by appointment to the public. At the PHM the curatorial and display work is undertaken by volunteers.

For General Audiences/Visitors

The responses of audiences and visitors to exhibitions and displays of the histories of mental health also shape the meanings of these collections. The exhibition A Closed World garnered widespread media attention; visitor numbers, including school groups, were steady, suggesting that curiosity about the 'closed world' of mental health was certainly present in the wider community.[42] Reactions to exhibitions elsewhere suggest that clients of the psychiatric system evince strong curiosity about the way that representations of past psychiatry are both constructed and received.[43] Although my research has not extended to audience and visitor perceptions of museum exhibitions, this is one direction such research should take so that we might better understand

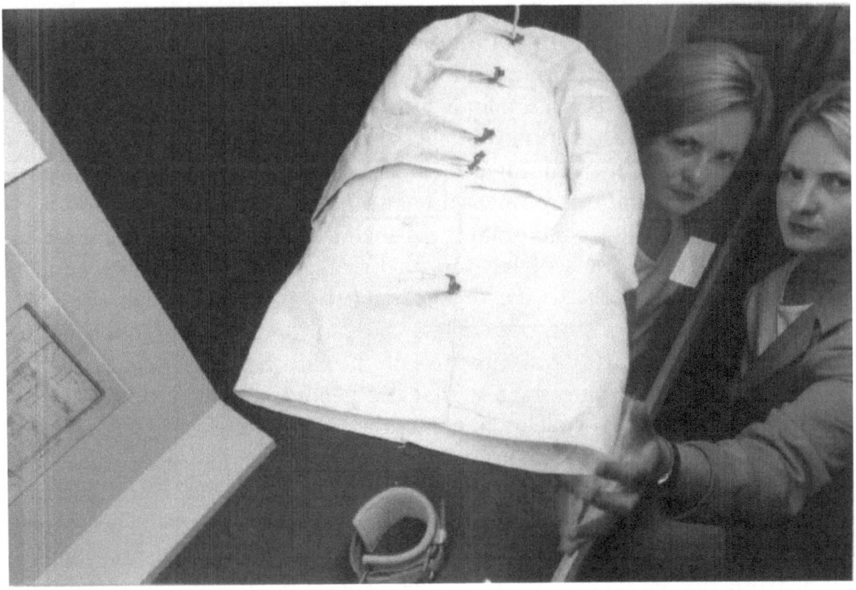

Figure 2.2 Catharine Coleborne poses beside a glass case exhibit of a straitjacket, January 1999.
Source: Courtesy of *The Age* newspaper, published 30 January 1999, p. 41. Reproduced with permission of Michael Rayner / Fairfax Photos.

the impacts and meanings of mental health collections and their display. In her chapter for this volume, Veis covers many of these points in more detail and from the perspective of a professional museum curator. In addition, Besley and Finnane show rich evidence of visitor engagement with the Remembering Goodna exhibition in their chapter.

HIDDEN OBJECTS AND THEIR PROVENANCE: SOME CONCLUSIONS

Objects and the role of 'things' in the lives of those hospitalized as insane have been relevant to public audiences before now, but for different reasons. In the nineteenth century, supporters of the hospitals for the insane sent gifts of fruit, magazines and newspapers, games, and other items to the patients. Such charitable giving reminds us of the significance of objects to patients and to the staff who cared for them. Yet these 'things' have been too readily overlooked. Bjørnar Olsen suggests that the material world has been forgotten by scholars, attributing this to the dominant philosophical trend of the twentieth century to reify textuality, and to the disavowal of the relationships forged between objects and people.[44] Olsen argues for objects as 'actors' in the drama of the narrative.[45] In the case of psychiatric collections, this approach might unfold a complex narrative of the relationships between things and people in institutional settings, as the chapter by Fiona R. Parrott in this volume indicates.

Material objects allow us new insights into a world of institutional histories shaped by an overwhelming wealth of written evidence. The privileging of textual representations of mental health has been inevitable given both the extent of official archival materials such as patient cases, and also the disciplinary expectations of written historical accounts and their status. Yet objects reveal more to us, provoking new questions about the past. These objects have been more or less 'hidden' to both scholars and the public until the institutional closures of the late twentieth century. The collections discussed here suggest that the peeling away of the many layers of interpretation of objects is necessary to fully explicate the cultural histories of confinement. The journeys taken by some objects are also part of their provenance and therefore the meanings produced by the collection. In the case of the Charles Brothers Collection, a small pharmacy was found at Ararat Mental Hospital, together with most of the collection's surgical instruments, while agricultural implements came from Beechworth and Sunbury. Most of the clothing was collected from Kew Mental Hospital, and an isolation cell was found by Dr Brothers sitting on an outside verandah.[46] The Mental Health Museum of WA was partly constructed from institutional objects, and patient casebooks containing a thousand cases were found dumped on a verandah at Lemnos Hospital in Perth on their way to local tip in 1995.[47] Their lonely, abandoned status before their collection pains their later champions and collectors. These odd collections of things have come to possess meaning through their interpretation as having a shared history of purpose and use across institutional sites.

Collections of psychiatric objects are also marginal within museological settings. For a long time, the Charles Brothers Collection, championed by its curator at the Museum of Victoria, was never exhibited. Large public museums have exhibited on medical themes to general audiences, such as the 'Mind and Body' and the 'Science of Life' galleries at the Melbourne Museum, Museum Victoria, in Melbourne's Exhibition Gardens. Successive curators documented ways that this collection might be exhibited, arguing for the importance of mental health to social history, the significance of specific commemorations in the late 1980s, as well as making links to genealogical practices and the work of family historians in using asylum records.[48] But the underlying problem, as curators themselves identify, is political: if mental health had a 'chequered history in Victoria', as it did elsewhere, the project to seek a 'balanced' perspective almost certainly means that more detailed and multi-faceted research needs to shape museum exhibitions for their different audiences.[49]

This chapter has set out some ways to understand the many collections of psychiatric objects in the late twentieth century through a series of discussions about their genesis, their collectors, aspects of their provenance, and briefly, their meanings for different users and audiences. Objects have lives beyond their display in exhibitions, and psychiatric collections also embody symbolic meanings, especially in an era of significant change to the mental health sector.

NOTES

1. Elizabeth Willis, "Home But Away: Material Evidence of Lives in Victorian Asylums, 1850–1950," *Psychiatry, Psychology and Law* 2, no. 2 (1995): 115.
2. Willis, "Home But Away", 115; see also Catharine Coleborne, *Reading 'Madness': Gender and Difference in the Colonial Asylum in Victoria, Australia, 1848–1880s*. Debut Book 2 (Perth: Network Books, 2007).
3. On the 'new social history', see Peter Burke, *What is Cultural History?* (Cambridge: Polity, 2008). See also Robert Berkhofer, *Fashioning History: Current Practices and Principles* (New York: Palgrave Macmillan, 2008), 155.
4. Roy Rosenzweig and David Thelen, *The Presence of the Past: Popular Uses of History in American Life* (New York: Columbia University Press, 1998).
5. One good example of this is the exhibition of Goodna Mental Hospital, Queensland at the Museum of Brisbane in 2007. The process of creating this exhibition is discussed further in this volume by Joanna Besley and Mark Finnane. See also Fiona Paisley, "Peeling Back History: The Remembering Goodna Exhibition", *Health and History* 11, no. 1 (2009): 172–178. An exhibition of the social history of Tokanui Hospital in New Zealand, titled Tokanui: Footprints on the Land, was held at the Te Awamutu Museum in 2006; see Michael Healy, "'No Easy Answer': Displaying Mental Health Histories in Local Museums," *Health and History* 9, no. 1 (2007): 149–153.
6. See Michael Healy's study of the online representation of mental health in museums, in which he assesses two museums with mental health exhibits developed online: "Digital Public History: How Small History Museums Are Using the Web," Unpublished Directed Study, History Programme, University of Waikato (2009).
7. In this chapter I draw upon several pieces of my own scholarly work to mount a new argument; see Catharine Coleborne, "Exhibiting 'Madness': Material Culture and the Asylum", *Health and History* 3, no. 2 (2001): 104–117; "Remembering Psychiatry's Past: The Psychiatric Collection and Its Display at Porirua Hospital Museum, New Zealand," *Journal of Material Culture* 8, no. 1 (2003): 97–118; and "Collecting 'Madness': Psychiatric Collections and the Museum in Victoria and Western Australia," in *'Madness' in Australia: Histories, Heritage and the Asylum,* ed. Catharine Coleborne and Dolly MacKinnon (St Lucia: University of Queensland Press, 2003), 183–189.
8. 'Making history' is a term deployed by a range of museum studies scholars; see for instance, Gaynor Kavanagh, *Making Histories in Museums* (London: Leicester University Press, 1996). On the 'material turn', see *Material Powers: History and the Material Turn,* ed. Tony Bennett and Patrick Joyce (London: Routledge, 2010).
9. Russell W. Belk, *Collecting in a Consumer Society.* Collecting Cultures (London: Routledge, 1995), 29–35; Sean Hides, "The Genealogy of Material Culture and Cultural Identity," in *Experiencing Material Culture in the Western World*, ed. Susan M. Pearce (London: Leicester University Press, 1997), 14–27. See also Ken Arnold, *Cabinets for the Curious: Looking Back*

at Early English Museums. Perspectives on Collecting (Aldershot: Ashgate, 2006).
10. Henrietta Riegel, "Into the Heart of Irony: Ethnographic Exhibitions and the Politics of Difference", in *Theorizing Museums: Representing Identity and Diversity in a Changing World,* ed. Sharon Macdonald and Gordon Fyfe. *Sociological Review* Monographs. (Oxford: Blackwell, 1996), 83–104.
11. Susan M. Pearce and Paul Martin, *The Collector's Voice: Critical Readings in the Practice of Collecting.* Vol. 4: Contemporary Voices. Perspectives on Collecting (Aldershot: Ashgate, 2002), xiii.
12. Belk, *Collecting in a Consumer Society,* 83–87.
13. Susan M. Pearce, "The Urge to Collect", in *Interpreting Objects and Collections* (London: Routledge, 1994), 157–159. See also the range of short essays in Pearce's edited volume.
14. On psychiatric institutions as heritage sites, see Martin R. Lipp, *Medical Landmarks USA: A Travel Guide* (New York: McGraw-Hill, 1991); Ray Osborne, "Asylums as Cultural Heritage: The Challenges of Adaptive Reuse," in Coleborne and MacKinnon, *'Madness' in Australia,* 217–229; Alun E. Joseph, Robin A. Kearns, and Graham Moon, "Recycling Former Psychiatric Hospitals in New Zealand: Echoes of Deinstitutionalisation and Restructuring", *Health & Place* 15, no. 1 (2009): 79–87.
15. Coleborne, "Remembering Psychiatry's Past," 10.
16. Ken Arnold, "Time Heals: Making History in Medical Museums," in Kavanagh, *Making Histories in Museums,* 15–29.
17. On medical networks, see M. Anne Crowther and Marguerite W. Dupree, *Medical Lives in the Age of Surgical Revolution* (Cambridge: Cambridge University Press, 2007).
18. Health and Medicine Museums Special Interest Group (HMM), *Guide to Health and Medicine Collections, Museums and Archives in NSW and ACT* (Sydney: Special Interest Group, 2003). A guide to New Zealand collections and museums also exists: http://archive.amol.org.au/hmm/about.html. See also the newsletter *The HaMMer* produced by the HMM, 1993–2005: http://archive.amol.org.au/hmm/back.htm.
19. W. D. Rubinstein and Hilary L. Rubinstein, *Menders of the Mind: A History of the Royal Australian and New Zealand College of Psychiatrists, 1946–1996* (Auckland: Oxford University Press, 1996), 14; Obituary, Charles Ronald David Brothers, *The Medical Journal of Australia,* 22 February 1964, 289–290.
20. Coleborne, "Collecting 'Madness'", 185–188.
21. Elizabeth Willis and Karen Twigg, *Behind Closed Doors: A Catalogue of Artefacts from Victorian Psychiatric Institutions Held at the Museum of Victoria* (Melbourne: Museum of Victoria, 1994).
22. Willis, "Home But Away", 111–116.
23. See Coleborne, "Collecting 'Madness'", 188–192.
24. See Coleborne, "Remembering Psychiatry's Past."
25. Information located in Museum Victoria records. The Kew Asylum Museum was opened in 1996, following the institutional closure in 1988. See also Daniel Cass and Lisa Cianci, *A Guide to the Records and Artefacts of the Kew Asylum Museum* (Melbourne: Australian Science Archives Project, 1996).
26. See Healy, "'No Easy Answer'."
27. Lipp, *Medical Landmarks USA.*
28. In New Zealand and Australia, public history has been developed by both scholars and practitioners. See for instance Graeme Davison, *The Use and Abuse of Australian History* (Sydney: Allen & Unwin, 2000); work by Paula

Hamilton and Paul Ashton, including their journal *Public History Australia*; and *Going Public: The Changing Face of New Zealand History*, ed. Bronwyn Dalley and Jock Phillips (Auckland: Auckland University Press, 2001). For built heritage, see note 14.

29. Anne Fahy asserts the notion of the 'primacy of the object' in the museum in her chapter "New Technologies for Museum Communication", in *Museum, Media, Message*, ed. Eilean Hooper-Greenhill (London: Routledge, 1999), 83. The idea of the object as a document of reality is taken from Ivo Maroevi , "The Museum Message: Between the Document and Information", in Hooper-Greenhill, 25–27.
30. Pearce, "Collecting as Medium and Message" in Hooper-Greenhill, 21–22.
31. Coleborne, "Remembering Psychiatry's Past," 112.
32. See Coleborne, "Collecting 'Madness'," 192–193.
33. Gaynor Kavanagh adopts Sheldon Annis' concept of 'dream space' as she articulates three 'spaces' across which museums operate: the cognitive, the social, and the dream space. Representations operate at the cognitive level, audiences move through the social space and also engage in collective and individual recognition and remembering work, and the dream space might be said to be a space for emotional responses and unconscious reactions to feed the interactions between museums and audiences/visitors. See Kavanagh, *Dream Spaces: Memory and the Museum* (London: Leicester University Press, 2000), 2–3; *Making Histories in Museums*, 1–14.
34. See Simon Cross, "Visualizing Madness: Mental Illness and Public Representation," *Television and New Media* 5, no. 3 (2004): 197–216.
35. Willis, "Home But Away", 111–112. The Brothers Collection is now part of the 'Medicine in Society Collection' at Museum Victoria.
36. Suzanne Hunt, "The Charles Brothers Mental Health Museum Collection Report," 1986. Museum of Victoria Research Library, Folder E, 1–2.
37. Willis, "Home But Away," 115.
38. Hunt, "The Charles Brothers Mental Health Museum Collection Report," 1986, 1.
39. Ibid., 3.
40. See Coleborne, "Exhibiting 'Madness'."
41. See Coleborne, "Collecting 'Madness'," 188–190.
42. I was interviewed for radio and television five times, including Radio National 621 ABC Breakfast, interview with Louise Adler. A newspaper article in the 'Health' pages, 'Lifting the lid on a system of madness', appeared in the *The Age*, 30 January 1999, 41.
43. Stephanie Lambert discusses the strong response from both former clients and staff to the exhibition of Tokanui's history in New Zealand in her chapter for a forthcoming collection about the histories of mental health in the Waikato region and Tokanui , 1912–2000. Publication details are not yet available, but this project is underway.
44. Bjørnar Olsen, "Material Culture After Text: Re-Membering Things," *Norwegian Archaeological Review* 36, no. 2 (2003): 94.
45. Olsen, 99.
46. Hunt, "The Charles Brothers Mental Health Museum Collection Report," 1986, 1.
47. Coleborne, "Collecting 'Madness'," 189.
48. Hunt, "The Charles Brothers Mental Health Museum Collection Report," 1986, 2.
49. Ibid., 3.

3 Pictures of People, Pictures of Places
Photography and the Asylum

Barbara Brookes

The great age of lunatic asylums—the nineteenth century—coincided with the development and rapid growth of photography. Today we have a photographic residue from the working asylums, including publicity photographs and postcards that show external panoramic views of their architectural splendor and interior photographs of clean wards and uniformed warders and starched nurses. Yet another interior archive exists from working asylums which was never meant for public display: the photographs of patients, and sometimes their bodily parts, taken to enhance medical knowledge of mental pathology. These archives, currently taking new life in books and online, serve to remember the history of psychiatry in different ways and it is an archive which, unbound from its original context, creates new meanings.

Photography offered a way to record individual sufferers of mental illness and such photographs were regarded as tools to assist with classification of illness. The scientific uses of the medium were quickly taken up, in places as diverse as New Zealand, Uruguay, Australia, the United States, and England, all of which will be discussed in this chapter. Photography's potential for reproduction allowed the circulation of images from asylums far beyond national borders, a potential exponentially increased today by the internet. Images of people, of body parts, or internal microscopic images of brain pathology might be used for medical training and to assist with diagnosis. These images form one kind of archive of the exploration of the external and internal working of the body and mind.

Apart from its scientific purposes, photography offered communities a way to advertise the grandeur of their civic buildings; an opportunity also grasped by private institutions. Panoramic vistas of grand buildings in extensive grounds depicted order and the progress of medical science in the treatment of the mentally ill. They captured a belief in the potential of the architecture, gardens, and surroundings themselves to have a therapeutic purpose. Photographs of orderly corridors and uniformed staff reinforced the perception that the asylum could provide respite for the ill. They reassured an anxious public that the institutions were sites of order. The grand buildings displayed civic pride and embodied the hope that the environment itself offered held a therapeutic promise.[1] They offer an archive intent on a narrative of progress.

In the twenty-first century the monumental abandoned asylums capture the imagination of urban explorers intent on exploring the unseen and off-limits parts of the urban environment, architects with an historical bent, heritage enthusiasts, and photographers with a range of interests. The digital world contains a plethora of images of these places that were once out of bounds to the general public. An archive of abandonment is in the process of creation, accessible through a web search on 'asylum photography'. As they decay, asylum buildings have taken on a new aesthetic as a testament of a time past when the mentally ill lived in closed communities. The ruins of a grand building, in the words of photographer Shaun O'Boyle, even when empty, 'carry their history with them'.[2] Twenty-first century photographic essays on the asylum are creating a new archive that make an aesthetic of decay that tells a particular history.

This chapter will address the photographs of the fragile people, the dismembered parts, and the solid buildings that serve as a means of remembering the nineteenth-century lunatic asylum. The photographs of the people are locked in time: the moment when they faced the camera. Asylum buildings, however, might be photographed many times over their life and continue to be photographed today as sites of memory. While we could think of the photographs of people in nineteenth-century casebooks, in Susan Sontag's words, as 'Melancholy Objects,'[3] given the reasons that inspired their creation, the passage of time creates the possibility that they become a treasured archive for historians as a catalogue of everyday people, domestic servants and labourers, people whose photographs do not usually enter the archive. Georges Didi-Huberman writes of the way mad women and men were photographed and how the photographs were used to create a typology.[4] I want to suggest that the elapse of time allows the photographs to be liberated from typology and may instead stand as a reminder of the individuality of the people who entered the asylum walls.[5]

My argument is that photographs of 'types' made in asylums in the nineteenth century can be released by time back to individuality: to show us the humanity of people who perhaps did not usually get to pose for a camera. They assist in remembering the suffering of individuals. In contrast, nineteenth-century photographs of asylum buildings often conceal more than they reveal. Twenty-first century photographs of asylum ruins might work to create a particular typology of suffering: buildings that appear to be haunted by fear and pain with little hint of the possibility of refuge or cure which some patients found within their walls.

PHOTOGRAPHY AND THE ASYLUM

The uses of photography for recording mental states began in England on the initiative of Dr Hugh W. Diamond, who had a great interest in photography.[6] In 1848 he became resident superintendent of the Female Department of the Surrey County Lunatic Asylum and in 1852 presented a series of photographic portraits of 'types of insanity' to a group in London. Four years later, Diamond read a paper to the Royal Society entitled "On the Application of Photography to the Physiognomic and Mental Phenomena of Insanity." For Diamond, photography surpassed the limitations of words to describe mental states by 'the silent but telling language of nature'. The picture, he claimed, 'speaks for itself with the most marked precision.'[7]

In 1859 *The Lancet*, a leading medical journal, remarked that 'Photography is so essentially the Art of Truth—and the representative of Truth in Art—that it would seem to be the essential means of reproducing all forms and structures of which science seeks for delineation.'[8] Doctors were encouraged to use cameras to record pathology. In the case of mental illness, Didi-Huberman writes of the 'spectacular evidence' gathered by the most famous nineteenth-century French neurologist, Jean-Martin Charcot.[9] Charcot became a leader in neurology and attracted students from all over the world to the Salpêtrière, the great Parisian general hospital for women.[10] A young Sigmund Freud was amongst the scores of medical students who flocked to the Salpêtrière to learn from Charcot about neurological disorders. Charcot's demonstrations of patients with hysterical symptoms were unforgettable experiences.[11]

Photography replicated both Charcot's demonstrations of states of madness and the assertion of the power of the doctor over the patient. The fleeting displays of patients that were available to students at the Salpêtrière were cast in a more lasting archive through photographs that remain available to us today. The highly significant *Iconographie photographique de la Salpêtrière*, a work concerned with the creation of typologies, was published in 1878.[12] Photography, for Charcot, 'was simultaneously an experimental procedure (a laboratory tool), a museological procedure (scientific archive), and a teaching procedure (a tool of transmission).'[13]

Photography promised to advance scientific understanding. In mental illness, it continued an older tradition of graphic representations of types of mental illness and contributed to the continuation of that tradition.[14] Photographs were used to create illustrations in textbooks for the education of practitioners. Michel Frizot has noted, 'Human physiognomy, in particular, was seen as the visual indicator of the emotions.'[15] But at the same time photography had a more prosaic use: it provided a record of patients. As institutions for the care of the mentally ill grew in size, a photograph attached to a patient's record assisted staff in identification, a practice begun by the police and elaborated under the direction of Alphonse Bertillon in the Paris Prefecture of Police from 1882. The rise of modern industrial societies, with the consequent development of state bureaucracies, led to new means of tracking individuals. Once invisible to the state, the image of everyday people could now be captured in a two-dimensional material object, kept in a state file, and used as a means of surveillance and control. Photographs became just one of the ways in which people were transformed into records for state purposes.[16]

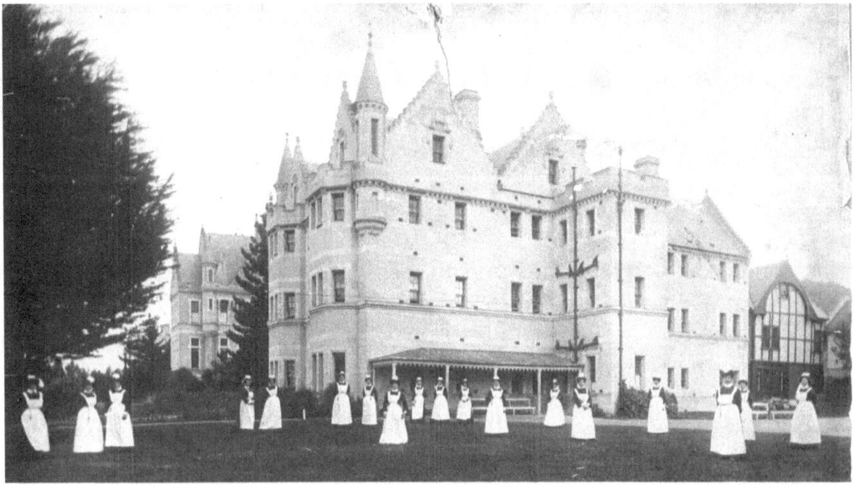

Figure 3.1 Nursing staff in front of Seacliff Asylum, circa 1890. DAHI/D266/2071/520a.
Source: Archives New Zealand/Te Rua Mahara o te Kāwanatanga, Dunedin Regional Office.

The technology that made such an archive possible, the camera, sometimes survives in collections. Frederic Truby King, Medical Superintendant of New Zealand's largest Lunatic asylum, Seacliff, from 1889 until 1921, was a keen photographer—as his requisitions ordering photographic supplies suggest.[17] Two of his cameras are now held in the collection of the New Zealand Centre for Photography. We do not know if it is the well-worn MIDG quarter plate camera, made between 1900 and 1910, which was used to take photographs of the asylum's patients.[18] Now, detached from its context, but slotted into the archive of photography, the work of the camera is difficult to recover. The date of the camera means it could not have been used to take the 1890 photograph of nurses on the lawn of the imposing asylum, outside Dunedin in southern New Zealand.

The image conveys the grandeur of the building and the cleanliness and order of the nursing staff. Such photographs can be found in a multitude of different asylum contexts worldwide. Communities were proud of the grand buildings erected to house the mentally ill 'that would serve as models of an enlightened society.'[19]

CAPTURED BIOGRAPHIES

A significant number of patients never left the great asylums and their photographs provide one vivid way into their lives: perhaps one of the few material traces they have left behind. The Burns Archive, New York, has accessioned albums entitled *Manicomio Departamento de Mujeres* (National Madhouse: Woman's Section) from the primary psychiatric facility at Montevideo, Uruguay. Photographs from these albums are reproduced in *Patients & Promise: A Photographic History of Mental and Mood Disorders.*[20] The photographs inspire our curiosity because they are of individuals captured in a context that suggests their distress. While the trained medical gaze may be able to detect a range of symptoms in the women who face the camera, to the lay person the portraits present women of different ages and moods whose stories cry out for more explication. What grief assails thirty-four-year-old Zuaria De M., admitted to the asylum on 20 September 1907? Of who or what is Eugenia A. thinking with her eyes closed and her pensive expression? What disease or accident led to the death of twenty-four-year-old Emilia D.? While these questions cannot be answered by the single photographs, the viewer feels a sense of closure in viewing the two images of sixteen-year-old Eva di L., the first at her entry to the asylum and the second as she left four months later. Here are documents that allow us to visualise a cross-section of Uruguayan women, and give us a sense of the cosmopolitan nature of that country.[21]

The *Patients and Promise* portraits are presented detached from the case notes, whereas asylum casebooks in many different national contexts capture the lives of people of varying ages, occupations and life experiences. At times the thin biographies in the case notes, varying according to the physical ailments and troublesomeness of patients, are brought to life by a photograph. The photographs, like those from Montevideo, are compelling because they are of people whose photographs may not have survived were they not captured in the asylum archive.

Three photographs of Johanna Becket are attached to her 1890 case file in the Seacliff Asylum archives. A forty-four-year-old married woman, her lined face speaks to a life of hard work. She had been in the asylum before and seemed perfectly aware of her surroundings, but was restless and anxious. Dr. Frederic Truby King, Superintendent of the asylum, wrote in his medical notes of her constant preoccupation with her hair. 'She ties her hair up & then shakes it all loose to do it up again in another way.' In a woman, disheveled hair signified a disordered mind. In the first of the three photographs, Johanna is seated and looks off to the side, distracted from the presence of the camera. Her hair is mostly down, while some appears caught at the top with a clip. In the second—and most compelling—photograph, Johanna stares intently at the camera from where she sits, her hands raised to her head, her hair flowing behind them. In both these photographs Johanna wears a pinafore over her striped dress. In the third photograph, we see a demure older woman standing, hands clasped before her, hair tightly tied in a bun on the top of her head. King validated use of the latter photograph as evidence, writing prior to Johanna's discharge after four months in the asylum, that she was 'quite normal, vide photo 3.'[22]

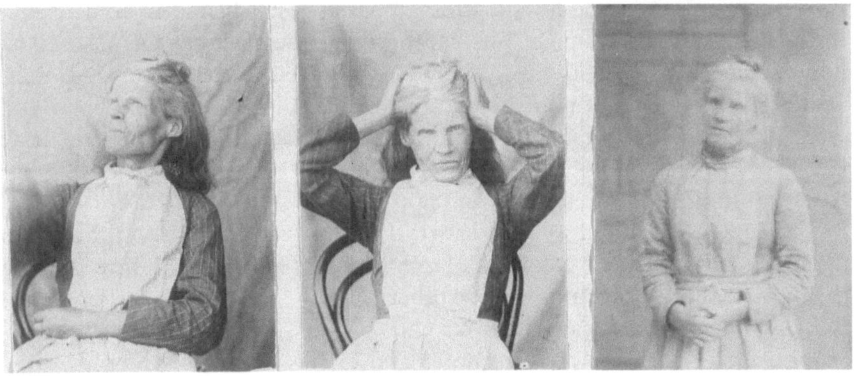

Figure 3.2 Johanna Beckett, DAHI/D264/19956/42.
Source: Archives New Zealand/Te Rua Mahara o te Kāwanatanga, Dunedin Regional Office.

A photograph taken in 1890 has the power to bring us face to face with a person who still challenges us. Johanna Beckett asks, "Why am I here? What is madness?" Indeed, she directly interrogated the man behind the camera, suggesting her awareness of both the performative nature of photography and the theatre of the clinic. She inquired of King in response to his request for a photograph: 'I suppose you want a picture of a madwoman. I'd better stick some straw in my hair and make faces.' Johanna Beckett knew the power of representation to reduce her individuality to a type. In the three images of Johanna that exist we can observe the creation of the very typology with which she was complicit; a typology which photography served to record and confirm. A progression of mental states is exactly what King attempted to capture in the three photographs.

The successive photographs of Johanna Beckett are unusual. Only a sample of the patients at Seacliff appears to have been photographed at this date and usually there is just a single image attached to the case file; a practice that we know occurred in other asylums.[23] The incidental nature of most of the photographs suggests that King, an amateur but keen photographer, was occasionally incorporating the camera into his clinical work. When there is an image, it is often pasted to the right of the personal information recorded in the specially printed, large, leather-bound casebooks.

The image lies beside the details of the patient's name, committal, sex, age, marital condition, occupation, religion and details of diagnosis. Sometimes the photographs are pasted elsewhere on the case notes and if there are multiple photographs, as in the case of Johanna, they are pasted on a sheet of lined paper inserted separately into the record. By 1896, however, there was a new level of professionalism in the photographic record. Just about every patient was photographed on admission. What was once a casual interest appears to have become routine.

We can only imagine how distressed patients felt being, in some cases, restrained while their image was captured for the asylum's purposes. The powerlessness of patients involuntarily committed to the asylum was replicated in the taking of their image for medical purposes of diagnosis and identification. It is our good fortune that we have an indication of how Johanna Beckett felt because Truby King was intrigued by her, finding her remarks 'smart and often witty and apropos.'

The images captured by medical staff and pasted in the Seacliff asylum files were not taken for any kind of exhibition. There is no indication that they were used for teaching (Didi-Huberman's 'tool of transmission') since they lay buried in the case files. We can assume, however, that the photographs, along with the medical notes and charts, informed doctors' decisions about patient care. At the very least, they allowed a mobile workforce of medical staff to recognize patients under their care.

In Johanna Beckett's exchange with Truby King, we get a glimpse of the patient side of the interaction. Perhaps patients were less passive subjects of the powerful doctor's gaze than we might imagine. Posing for the doctor's camera made them the object of special attention; some may have resented it, and required restraint, others may have welcomed it, and even requested that a portrait be made.

Whatever bargains were made in interposing the camera between doctor and patient, what was recorded has the power to restore to today's viewer the humanity of the mentally ill in the way that the written text rarely can. We see a captured moment of the past, which in turn becomes a reminder of our own mortality.[24] While the case note described 'a small thin wiry woman with a very fair complexion & hair (tending to albino)', the photograph conveys a direct, serious, and enquiring gaze. This, the photograph suggests, is not a woman to be trifled with.

Case notes were written by staff who observed and interpreted the moods of patients. From intercepted letters, pasted into the files, we sometimes get the words of patients themselves, but these are rare. The photographs bring us face to face with nineteenth-century working people, labourers and domestic servants, whose lives have taken a turn for the worse. We view these photographs in the knowledge that they were generated at a time when mental illness led to incarceration. While doctors may have photographed patients in an attempt to create typologies of mental illness, the captured portraits in the archive do the opposite today. They resurrect individuals in all their particularity. Johanna Beckett's direct gaze reminds us of the thin line between her state and ours.

PHOTOGRAPHY IN THE LABORATORY: THE FRIERN ASYLUM ALBUM

Europe's largest 'Italianate Style' asylum, the Middlesex County Pauper Lunatic Asylum at Colney Hatch, opened with pomp and ceremony in

1851. Only a three-part panorama photograph could capture the extent and magnificence of the building at the time of its opening since it initially covered some 118 acres and had six miles of corridors.[25] Initially the large and imposing asylum held 1,250 patients, already a daunting number to record. By 1937, when it was renamed Friern Hospital, the institution held 2,700 patients. This large hospital closed in 1995.

An album of photographs taken at Colney Hatch between 1890 and 1910 survives because a relative of the doctor who compiled it gave it to the last medical superintendant of the hospital. He in turn passed it to Richard Hunter who, together with Ida Macalpine, wrote a history of the hospital, *Psychiatry for the Poor,* published in 1974.[26] The album is a collage that challenges the viewer to make sense of the layout and individual photographs. Photographs of brain sections sit alongside photographs of people in the album held in the Wellcome Collections. A couple of its pages are viewable online.[27]

By the time of the composition of the Friern album, the brain was the place where the problems of the asylum's inmates were thought to reside. In the interior recesses of the brain lay disturbances that resonated throughout the body.[28] Research on the brain was proceeding apace and those working in the field might keep wet samples or brain slices. Photographs, however, offered a much easier form of evidence both to keep and to circulate amongst colleagues. On pages of the album there are prints of parts of more than one brain, presented in various sections, in the hope that the images might reveal the malady of the sufferer to the medical expert who appraised them and inserted them into the collection. Hunter and Macalpine describe the pathological states that some of the photographs in the album illustrate.[29] In these images we see the use of photography, in Didi-Huberman's words, as 'an experimental procedure' or a 'laboratory tool'.

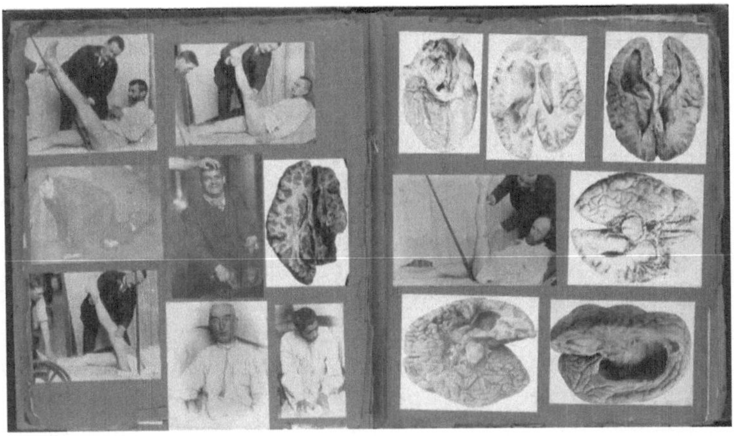

Figure 3.3 L0063567, Friern Hospital Album, Friern Barnet, 1890–1910, p.14. *Source*: Wellcome Library, London.

Chance determined the survival of this album, and its accession by the Wellcome. Within the album's covers lie photographs of deformed feet, noses and sexual organs, cadavers, petri dishes with organisms, naked and clothed people, people with skin ravaged by spots and splotches and, every now and then, a shy face smiling at the camera. These are photographs that attempt to dissect madness and make its features apparent to the medical gaze. While in this case these images were pasted into an album, other photographs of unusual cases were exchanged by doctors in medical networks that extended across Britain, North America, South Africa, India, Australia and New Zealand.[30]

The occasional patient in the Friern album looks back at us from the late nineteenth century. How do we read the expression on the face of the man whose legs have been amputated? Is it a smile or a grimace? His hands and fingers draw our attention to the stumps of his legs. Is the hand on his head necessary to steady him or to ensure that he faces the camera? Is the person touching or holding him engaged in care or coercion? Amongst the many questions it raises this photograph firmly reminds us that asylums provided care for the physical, as well as the psychiatric, needs of patients. Here was a man who perhaps needed more care than was available for the poor outside of an institution.

RE-ENVISAGING THE ASYLUM AND ITS INHABITANTS

Over the course of its history, the original asylum at Colney Hatch changed its name many times in order to cast off unwanted associations.[31] Old photographs take on a new life on YouTube and we can view of history of the asylum under its current name, Princess Park Manor.[32] The former asylum has now been refurbished by developers into 260 luxury apartments with a health club attached.[33]

The developers' Princess Park Manor website gives us the date of the conception of the building and we are told that 39 leading architects vied to design it. We are not told that they were designing an asylum, rather that it was 'A Victorian Masterpiece which has delighted and inspired aficionados of fine architecture for generations.' Whereas once security was designed to keep inmates in, the current 24-hour manned security gate and CCTV are designed to keep the public out of the exclusive world of apartment owners and their 'state of the art health and fitness club.'[34] This new visual representation of the asylum works to eradicate its history.

There are, however, alternative histories on screen. In 1998, Rebecca Frayn made a documentary for Channel 4's Cutting Edge entitled 'Asylum' which brought together former patients and future residents.[35] One new resident confides she had been 'feeling pretty suicidal before she moved in' and hopes that Princess Park Manor will 'bring her new friends and romances.' 'How ironic', the presenter commented, 'that people are now willing to pay large sums of money to live in a place that advertises itself as somewhere "you never need to leave".'[36] While once families with resources might pay vast sums for the seclusion of their mentally ill relatives in private asylums, individuals can now choose to buy such seclusion for themselves in the former public asylum's apartments and adjoining health club.

Not only buildings, but also patients, can be re-envisaged. The Australian photographer Anne Ferran has reworked the photographs of thirty-eight female psychiatric patients taken in the Sydney hospital in the 1940s. In keeping with the desire of many who preserve the psychiatric archive to protect the anonymity of the patients, Ferran shows sections of the body or, through layering the faces, produces 'a kind of invisibility.' A commentator notes that 'it is characteristic of Ferran's work that the subject is not is what is seen in the photograph but something only partly visible which haunts it.'[37] This work was exhibited at the Stills Gallery, Sydney, in 2003 and some of it can be viewed online.

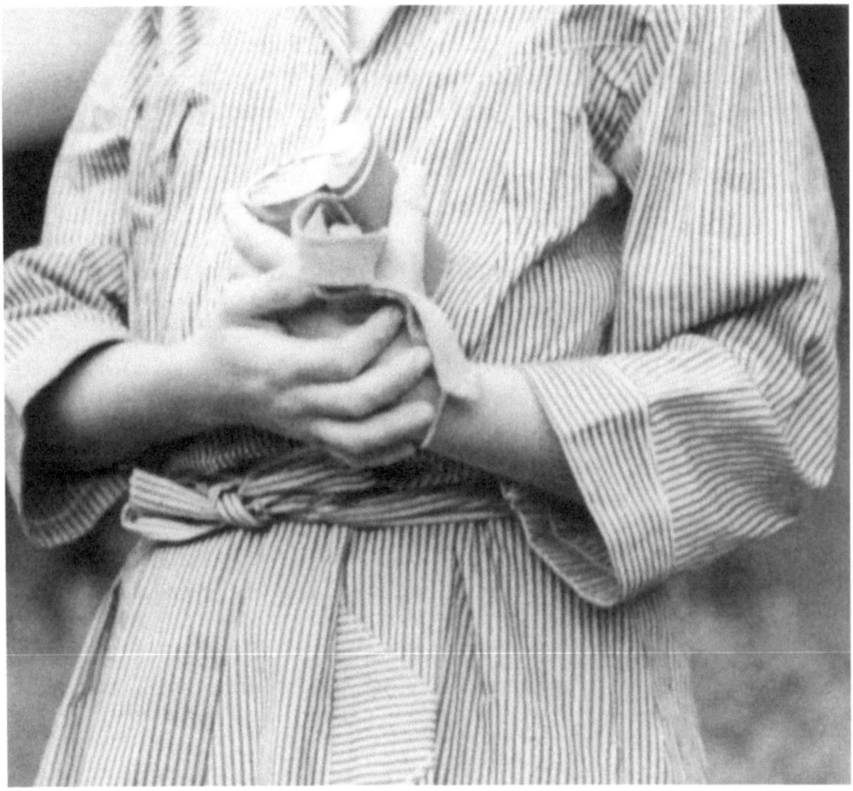

Figure 3.4 Anne Ferran: Image 4, 2003, '1–38' Series, Stills Gallery website.
Source: Courtesy of Anne Ferran.

PHOTOGRAPHIC ELEGIES

The initial community pride in grand asylum buildings, like the Seacliff Asylum that became Johanna Beckett's home, faded as the buildings themselves aged and sensibilities changed. When the move to deinstitutionalisation gained ground in the 1960s, the old buildings came to stand for a discredited past regime. In the twenty-first century, however, the abandoned buildings without inhabitants, but with an imagined past, have been imbued with a new aesthetic value in books and in online photographic essays. Details of beautifully crafted items such as door knobs, elegant radiators and Italianate water towers make us aware of a time when public buildings were more than simply utilitarian. But the incongruity of the isolated objects challenges the viewer. How are we to interpret the butter knife left on a window ledge or the x-ray in a window?[38] A sense of estrangement distances the world of the mentally ill from the world we inhabit. We may also feel troubled 'by the way photography inexorably beautifies';[39] how a photographic essay on a place once filled with the sadness of individuals can render the spaces serene and captivating.

Heidi Johnson's book *Angels in the Architecture* began as a commitment to document the significant architecture of the Northern Michigan Asylum which opened in 1885 and closed, by then named the Traverse City Regional Psychiatric Hospital, in 1989. The introductory essay by historian Nancy Tomes discusses the years from the mid-nineteenth century, when the idea of a therapeutic landscape held sway. Johnson goes on to introduce us to that landscape through the use of historical exterior and interior black and white photographs and her own photographs of surviving spaces. In this work an historical archive is skillfully blended with a new photographic record.

Johnson's photographs have black borders, suggesting both mourning and the depth and weight of old photographs printed on card. The photographs are often juxtaposed with recollections from people who worked at the hospital, from former patients, and documents relating to the institution, including case notes. The modern photographs work with the text to give insight into the daily life of a hospital that, over its existence, housed 50,000 patients, employed approximately 20,000 staff and welcomed over 250,000 visitors.[40] The sharpness of the historical photographs contrast with Johnson's images, which are sometimes shot with a dream-like, suffused light. Her final image records a patient's painting 'Forever': a head with pictograms rather like a phrenology model and underneath, the words:

> Remember
> Each Book you Read
> Each thot [*sic*] you Think
> Each Deed you do—is:

Henceforth Recorded
–Forever–
on the huge tape we call our
subconscious
Be ever so careful what you
Record[41]

This warning, painted on a support column in the basement of the women's cottage at the Traverse asylum and initially meant for other inmates, has now moved outside the basement and circulated the world through Heidi Johnson's photograph, available in the book and accessible online.[42] The photograph records an often ephemeral aspect of the psychiatric archive: patient graffiti.

Christopher Payne, an architect and photographer, spent six years documenting the fine facades and crumbling interiors of state mental hospitals in the United States. Payne's work recalls William Fox Talbot's 1830s observation of 'the camera's special aptitude for recording the "injuries of time."'[43] *Asylum: Inside the Closed World of State Mental Hospitals* (2009) is a visually stunning book. In many ways it is a book about absence. In the interior scenes of decay we see the array of gym shoes that people once wore, the neat coloured rows of toothbrushes once used, the pile of discarded packs of green *Salem* cigarettes once smoked, and coloured straitjackets: all have a pleasing, if disturbing, colour and symmetry. With the eye of an artist, Payne makes us see a beauty in the peeling paint, metal mesh doors and decaying utilitarian equipment. At first we first find the wooden framed collection of brightly coloured toothbrushes visually attractive but a closer look reveals the name labels that make us think of the people who used them. This intimate picture reveals the abandonment of personal privacy in the institutional setting.

Payne aimed to capture the scale and self-sufficiency of the large American state asylums by photographing the remaining parts of many to give a composite picture. The self-sufficiency of asylums relied on patient labour and many took pride and found meaning in their work.[44] Payne records this work in images such as the one of the shoe-making shop.

Here is a visual record of both the human needs and the human labour so central to maintaining the asylum communities. Other needs were clearly catered for as the images of art works, the barbershop, the hairdressing salon, the concert auditoriums, film projection equipment, the outdoor grandstand, the bowling alley, gymnasium and café suggest. Logansport State Hospital even boasted a TV studio.

Payne presents worlds unto themselves, whether the subterranean view of massive heating ducts and vast signposted underground passages or the sterile operating suite and tiered autopsy theatre. He does not shy away from death. Caskets, grave markers and cremation urns stand as a stark reminder that many of the inhabitants of asylums never left. This was their world.

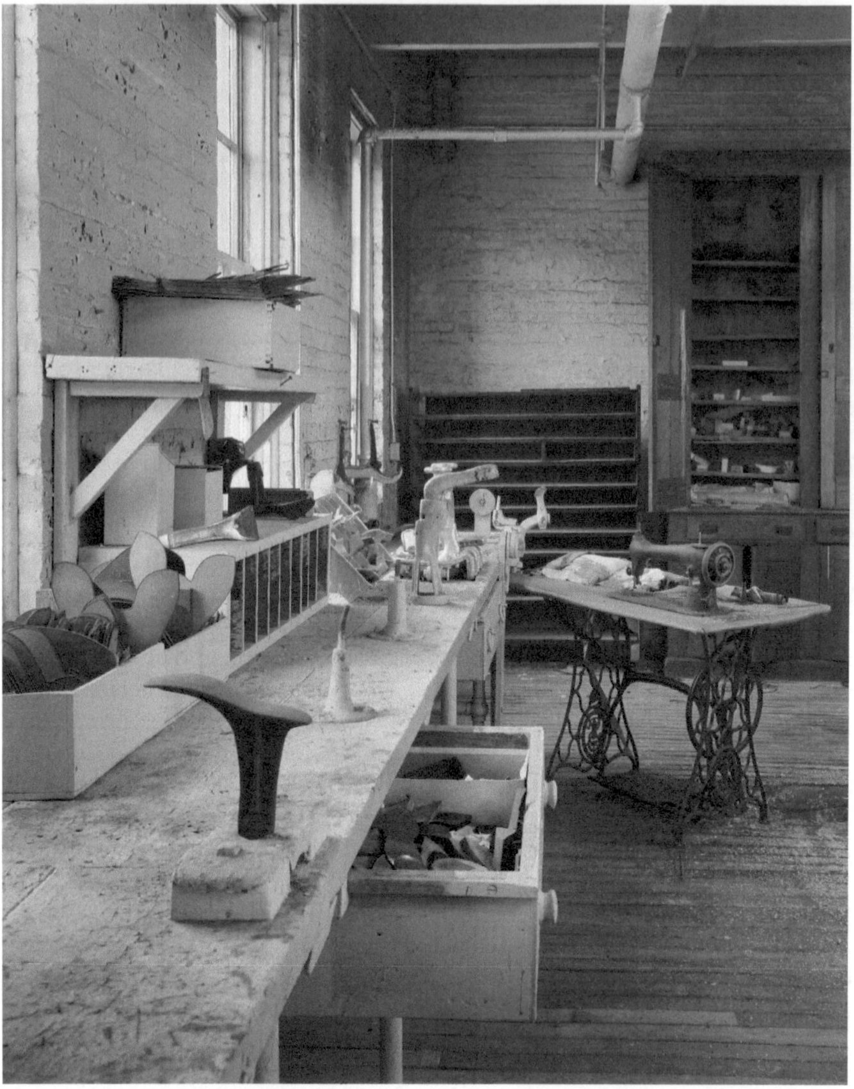

Figure 3.5 Christopher Payne, Shoe Shop, Taunton State Hospital.
Source: Christopher Payne, *Asylum: Inside the Closed World of State Mental Hospitals*, The MIT Press, p. 148.

The photographs of vast interior emptiness and decay suggest large-scale human suffering. Oliver Sachs, in his foreword to Payne's photographic narrative, relates an individual story that counters the visual tale of abandonment. Anna Agnew, he writes, committed to the Indiana Hospital for the Insane in 1878, 'felt profound relief when the institution closed protectively around her.' Unable to control her drive to harm herself and her children, Anna found that after a few days in the asylum:

> I felt a greater degree of contentment than I had felt for a year previous. Not that I was reconciled to life, but because my unhappy condition of mind was understood, and I was treated accordingly . . . I . . . was treated as an insane woman, a kindness not hitherto shown to me.[45]

While the photographs devoid of people hint of emptiness and despair, Anna Agnew's story suggests the protective shell that the asylum could provide.

It is the shell of the asylums that are the focus of Shaun O'Boyle's online photographs of state mental hospitals at Northampton, Utica, Buffalo and Byberry. O'Boyle's interest is in ruins and that is what these somber black and white images reveal. In his online flash movie, accompanied by the music of Phillip Glass, O'Boyle's coloured photographs show spaces of grand proportions and impressive architecture, sweeping staircases and fan- light windows, often flooded with natural light through the now open doors.[46] The empty hangers and unkempt beds remind us of the people who once were behind the closed doors of the grand buildings. The sequence ends with a photograph of an Algernon Charles Swinburne poem scratched on the wall of the lock up ward at a state asylum. The image makes the ephemeral permanent and, through words, recreates the mood of the patient who inscribed it:

> From too much love of living
> From hope and fear set free
> We thank with brief thanksgiving
> Whatever Gods may be
> That no man lives forever
> That dead men rise up never
> That even the weariest river
> Winds somewhere safe to sea.

O'Boyle's movie is a meditation upon the emptiness and decay of the asylum and how it recalls the past residents.[47]

Thomas Ryan, another photographer, records in detail the long history (1827–2000) of the Royal Derwent Hospital, Australia's oldest mental hospital. This visual record of 101 images captures the changing architectural styles that housed the mentally ill from the stately 1830s, the decorative art deco of the 1930s to the utilitarian 1970s. The graffitied and vandalised buildings include nurses' accommodation and a modernist church. The title 'Abandoned and Derilict [*sic*] Building Study' might gesture towards the way in which viewers are to remember the inhabitants. This is a serious visual history with the architecture at its centre, annotated at times with notes about the buildings portrayed.[48] The enclosed exercise yards stand as a reminder of the restraints on those who lived within the hospital's walls.

A very different memorial is the 'Abandoned Mental Asylum Hellingly, RIP, 33 Creepy Photo Tribute', an online urban explorers' record of their daring visit to the 'rotten bedlam of massive Hellingly Asylum' in Sussex built in 1903 and closed in 1994. The authors of the work note that the asylum is to be replaced with new housing and offer good luck to those 'who think you will live peacefully on land soaked with trauma.'[49] Viewers are invited 'to go off the rails' to explore the 'decomposing mental hospital' that once had its own railway and which is now in the process of being torn down. The photographs of interior decay reveal weather damage, vandalism, arson and graffiti. Unlike the seriousness of many other photographic records, there is playfulness in this memorialisation that puns on the abandonment of the mentally ill, just as the buildings are now abandoned. Tricks of photography allow the merging of the old and the new as a black and white image of a ward in its heyday is merged with the dilapidated bathroom graffitied with the image of a nude arising from the bath. The Tribute ends with a photo of 'ghosts': a particular and perhaps apt reminder that once these cavernous and decaying rooms were peopled.

The out-of-kilter world of the mentally ill is captured most powerfully in further photographs of Hellingly from DeviantArt, an online art community founded in 2000.[50] The Hellingly photographs are taken at angles that tip corridors on their sides, foreground holes in the floor into which the unwary might tumble, and suggest the 'crazy choices' of branching corridors. In the world of 'deviant' photographers, nature reasserts itself and chaos abounds in the derelict buildings that have become the haunt of graffiti artists and seekers after scary thrills.[51] This digital photography delights in chaos, in contrast to the measured and calm appraisal evident in Payne's record of asylums.

CONCLUSION

The photographer, Susan Sontag writes, 'both loots and preserves, denounces and consecrates'.[52] The medical men who photographed the brains of patients robbed the dead of images for medical purposes. Yet those images can now serve to memorialise a time when knowledge of the brain was transformed by photographic images that could be readily exchanged. Photography was put to the service of science in recording the lesions in the brain that were the footprint of a lifetime of suffering. It became a 'laboratory tool' and a 'scientific archive' for neurologists and psychiatrists in their quest to unravel the mind's mysteries. The Friern Album reminds us of the inseparability of the brain from the body, of the organs from personhood. People, body parts, and petri dishes jumbled together suggest the indivisibility of asylum life, where scientific investigation and daily regimes of work and care all took place.

Old asylum buildings are often imagined to have ghosts: the spirits of those poor souls condemned to a hell on earth. People seeking the glamour of the architecture—or the adventure of exploring a once inaccessible and now forbidden site—put the buildings to new uses. Through photography, then, some of these visitors are creating a new archive. Photographs of asylum buildings remind us of the sheer size of the institutional communities and their self-sufficient nature. Their architectural grandeur speaks to a pride of investment in public buildings. At the same time, their monumental size and current emptiness can stand as a rebuke for past values that may appear inhumane. Photographs of decay serve to denounce an earlier regime.

When we view the photographs of individual patients, however, and read the casebooks, we can see that asylums provided a sense of refuge for some, a short respite from the demands of the world for others, and for many, a final home. Lives that are absent in the photographs of empty and abandoned buildings can be made legible through creative interweaving of oral history, documentary sources, historical and contemporary photographs. The photographic archive, enriched by case notes, allows us to piece together the vicissitudes of life that led to committal to the asylum. Photographs of people once taken to record an instance of 'mania' or 'cerebral dementia', for example, when released from the medical context of their making, suggest ordinary lives caught in a particular moment. If we can record these lives and place the extraordinary fact of asylum committal in the mundane world of everyday citizens, then the photographic archive can assist in restoring the humanity of the mentally ill and remind us that we could well share their fate.

NOTES

1. Nancy Tomes, "The Asylum as Therapeutic Landscape," in Johnson, *Angels in the Architecture: A Photographic Elegy to an American Asylum*, ed. Heidi Johnson, Great Lakes Books (Detroit: Wayne State University Press, 2001), 1–18.
2. http://oboylephoto.com/ruins/intro.htm (accessed December 7, 2010).
3. Susan Sontag, *On Photography* (Harmondsworth: Penguin, 1979), 49.
4. Georges Didi-Huberman, *Invention of Hysteria: Charcot and the Photographic Iconography of the Salpêtrière*, trans. Alisa Hartz (Cambridge, MA: MIT Press, 2003, 29–66.
5. Dolly MacKinnon notes an example from a Scottish asylum where a patient wrote to Dr Thomas Clouston and included a photograph of himself in which he was at great pains to show his individuality and that the move to a different asylum would improve his treatment. Personal communication.
6. Sander L. Gilman, ed., *The Face of Madness: Hugh W. Diamond and the Origin of Psychiatric Photography* (New York: Brunner/Mazel, 1976), 6.
7. Hugh W. Diamond, "On the Application of Photography to the Physiognomic and Mental Phenomena of Insanity," paper read before the Royal Society, 22 May 1856, reprinted in Gilman, *Face of Madness*, 19.
8. Daniel M. Fox and Christopher Lawrence, *Photographing Medicine: Images and Power in Britain and America since 1840* (New York: Greenwood Press, 1988), 21.
9. Didi-Huberman, *Invention of Hysteria.*
10. Ibid., 13.

11. Mary King, *Truby King: The Man* (London: George Allen and Unwin, 1948), 41.
12. D. M. Bourneville and P. Regnard, *Iconographie Photographique de la Salpêtrière* (Paris: Progrès Médical/Delahaye, 1878).
13. Didi-Huberman, *Invention of Hysteria*, 30.
14. Emma Verry, "The Exposure of Truth: The Use of Photography in Mental Health in the Late Nineteenth and Early Twentieth Century," BA Hons. Diss., University of Otago, 2009, 13–30.
15. Michel Frizot, "Body of Evidence: The Ethnophotography of Difference," in *A New History of Photography*, ed. Michel Frizot (Cologne: Könemann, 1998), 260.
16. John Tagg, *The Disciplinary Frame: Photographic Truths and the Capture of Meaning* (Minneapolis: University of Minnesota Press, 2009); Michel Foucault, *Discipline and Punish: The Birth of the Prison*, trans. Alan Sheridan (London: Penguin, 1991), 191–192.
17. Verry, "The Exposure of Truth," 37.
18. NewZealandCentreforPhotography,http://www.nzcp.com/Features/tabid/122/articleType/ArticleView/articleld/40/Historic-Cameras-Truby-King-and-Ed-Hillary.aspx accessed April 1, 2011.
19. Christopher Payne, "The State Mental Hospitals: Their Origin, Construction, and Demise," in *Asylum: Inside the Closed World of State Mental Hospitals*, ed. Christopher Payne (Cambridge, MA: MIT Press, 2009), 7.
20. Stanley B. Burns, *Patients & Promise: A Photographic History of Mental and Mood Disorders. Seeing Insanity: Selections from the Burns Archive, 1845–1945* (New York: Burns Archive Press, 2006).
21. Six of the thirty-four women are described as Italian and one as a Brazilian.
22. Seacliff Lunatic Asylum—DAHI/19956/D264/42—2397—Medical Casebook entry for Patient 2397 (dated 1890–1891), Archives New Zealand/Te Rua Mahara o te Kāwanatanga, Dunedin Regional Office (hereafter ANZD).
23. Of the 97 patient files in the 1890–1891 Seacliff casebook, only thirty-three have photographs. Verry, "The Exposure of Truth," 37.
24. Roland Barthes, *Camera Lucida: Reflections on Photography*, trans. Richard Howard (London: Flamingo, 1984).
25. The panorama is reproduced in Richard Hunter and Ida Macalpine, *Psychiatry for the Poor: 1851 Colney Hatch Asylum—Friern Hospital 1973: A Medical and Social History* (Folkestone: Dawsons, 1974), 14–15.
26. Handwritten note by Richard Hunter, Folio 2. Wellcome Library, London.
27. http://images.wellcome.ac.uk/
28. Dr Thomas S. Clouston, James Middlemass and W. F. Robertson, "On the Typical Microscopic Lesions found in the Brain in Insanity: A Demonstration," *Journal of Mental Science* 40 (1894): 665–670.
29. Hunter and Macalpine, *Psychiatry for the Poor*, 240–245.
30. Personal communication, Dolly MacKinnon.
31. http://www.barnet.gov.uk/index/leisure-culture/libraries/archives/archives-histories/archives-finchleyhistories/archives-finchley-colneyhatchasylum.htm (accessed July 30, 2010).
32. http://www.youtube.com/watch?v=n_khf14rLPA accessed April 7, 2011.
33. Ray Osborne, "Asylums as Cultural Heritage: The Challenges of Adaptive Re-Use," in Coleborne and MacKinnon, *'Madness' in Australia*, 217–229.
34. http://www.princessparkmanor.net accessed April 7, 2011.
35. Brian Viner, "Television: Our Friends off the North Circular," *The Independent*, 14 March, 1999.
36. Eve Blake, "Visiting the Asylum," *London Review of Books*, 6 May, 2003.

37. http://www.stillsgallery.com.au/artists/ferran/index.php?obj_id=about&nav=0 accessed April 7, 2011.
38. Johnson, *Angels in the Architecture*, 121, 135.
39. Sontag, 107.
40. Johnson, *Angels in the Architecture*, 19.
41. Ibid., 187.
42. http://photo.net/photodb/photo?photo_id=1135402 accessed April 7, 2011.
43. Sontag, 69.
44. Oliver Sachs, "Asylum," in Payne, *Asylum: Inside*, 4.
45. Sachs, "Asylum," 1.
46. Sean O'Boyle, http://www.oboylephoto.com/state_hospital/sh_Movie2.htm accessed April 7, 2011.
47. O'Boyle, 'Modern Ruins,' http://oboylephoto.com/ruins/intro.htm accessed April 7, 2011.
48. Thomas Ryan, http://www.tryanphotos.com/Architecture/Abandoned-Derelict-Building/Royal-Derwent-Hospital/6417343_dQtDw#542924346_XsmpU accessed April 7, 2011.
49. http://weburbanist.com/2010/03/10/abandoned-mental-asylum-hellingly-rip-33-creepy-photo-tribute/ accessed April 7, 2011.
50. http://help.deviantart.com/116/ accessed April 7, 2011.
51. http://www.smashingshare.com/2010/06/09/hellingly-asylum-mental-hospital-photos/ accessed April 7, 2011.
52. Sontag, 54–55.

4 The Ethics of Exhibiting Psychiatric Materials

Nurin Veis

Any display of psychiatric collections should automatically observe ethical museum practice. This chapter looks first at the display of medical collections, and then focuses specifically on psychiatric collections within a museum context. Within this discussion, and because of the nature of these types of collections, I also draw parallels with the ethical issues associated with displaying human remains as well as diversity and disability collections. Writing as a museum curator, with over ten years of experience working with Museum Victoria's medical collection, I have first-hand knowledge of the difficulties such collections present. I explore the relevance of the museum's role in the ethical display of medical and psychiatric objects/collections, and comment on visitor reactions to, and expectations of such displays, as well as outlining specific issues that need to be addressed.

THE WONDER OF MEDICAL COLLECTIONS

Medical collections are often bizarre and confronting, yet many people find aspects of them intriguingly compelling.[1] Essentially, medical collections consist of objects that range from anatomical specimens, professional scientific instruments used in the practice of medicine and medical research, as well as artefacts ranging from items of domestic medicine to public health education. These objects have the potential to tell stories from various cultural perspectives, and different eras. Visitors are captivated by the gothic theatricality evoked by displays of medical artefacts whether they are anatomical specimens, obstetric instruments or a post mortem kit.[2] Medical exhibition audiences have a fascination with the unknown, the hidden, and at times, the forbidden. These medical collections can evoke in audiences dramatic experiences of high emotion—ranging from moments of pain and revulsion, recognition of stigma, as well as personal insight.

Medicine intersects with the worlds of science, technology, culture and ethics. As a consequence 'medicine', and its associated collections and their display, triggers questions about shared social values and issues of morality that relate to bodily practices. Medicine has the capacity to touch on many areas of public dialogue including issues of gender, conceptions of normality, and changing views on health and wellbeing, life and death. In all parts of the world there are impassioned debates surrounding the topics of contraception, abortion, and euthanasia.[3]

WHY DO WE DISPLAY MEDICAL COLLECTIONS?

Historically, the main purpose of medical collection displays in public museums is to tell public health stories of science and medicine, with the aim of informing the visitor about ways to improve their health and well-being. The most common approach has been to provide thematic, individual narratives on health. These collections have also traditionally told stories of the evolution of medical history that highlight issues of past medical practice, signalling how such practices might inform future change. Medical exhibitions are generally aimed at the broad general public, but they have also been targeted to specialist education audiences ranging from primary to tertiary students. Since the late twentieth-century medical displays have been much more open in their approach, incorporating themes of fine art, museology, philosophy and ethics. They often explore a multitude of issues concerning the body, the mind and medicine, examining both the past as

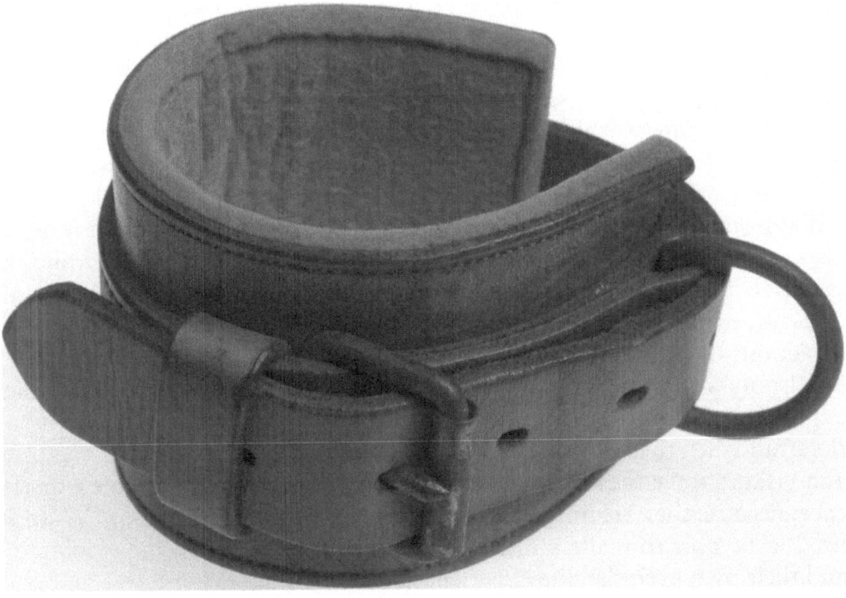

Figure 4.1 Wrist shackle used for restraining patients in a psychiatric hospital in Victoria, Australia, circa 1920.
Source: Photo by Jon Augier, Museum Victoria, Victoria, Australia.

well as projecting views on the future. Successful medical exhibitions strive to achieve both a strong emotional and intellectual connection with the visitor. An intellectually engaging exhibition may momentarily intrigue the visitor, but essentially fails to make a lasting impression unless it captures the imagination and resonates with a person's experience of life.

WHAT DO VISITORS EXPECT OF MEDICAL COLLECTION DISPLAYS?

Museum Victoria's audience research, conducted regularly over the period 1998–2007, has revealed that visitors entering a medical collection exhibition expect scientific information that is communicated in a clear and concise way. Any contemporary medical content should be directly relevant to issues of personal health, and should aim at assisting visitors to make informed choices about their health. Museum visitors expect the information to be accurate, interpreted, and contextualised within a broader framework; they also expect that the information contained in the display is trustworthy and presented without bias. If a specific interpretive stance is taken by the museum then it should be stated upfront and explicitly. Visitors expect the information to be authoritative without being condescending and autocratic.

Visitors are not empty vessels waiting to be filled with knowledge, but bring with them rich life experiences. They come with their own values and beliefs. Certain aspects of a medical exhibition, however, may be too confronting or controversial for a specific individual on any particular day. The visitor's choice to either stay or leave an exhibition must be valued. Therefore, appropriate warning signage at the entrance of any display must be exhibited, clearly stating that an exhibition's content may be controversial and might cause some visitors distress. The publicity for the exhibition and any information included on advertising fliers about the exhibition must also inform the reader or viewer that the display does contain confronting material. Themes that regularly challenge many visitors include anatomical displays, exhibitions about sex and sexuality, contraception, abortion and depictions of pain, illness, surgery, death and mental illness.

Visitors anticipate that any exhibition will be a special and intriguing experience that engages them both intellectually and emotionally. Exhibitions fail when they do not establish an emotional connection with visitors, and visitors leave these displays without any sense of a memorable experience, because they are unmoved by exclusively factual information. Visitors need to be able to make a meaningful correlation between the exhibition and their own everyday life experiences when visiting exhibitions.

Museum visitors expect to see authentic objects in exhibitions, and they are disappointed if reproductions are displayed. Reproductions and mock-ups must be clearly labelled as such, and, if possible, avoided. The community expects museums to deliver genuine experiences and a failure to do so undermines the visitors' expectation of museums as places of legitimacy.

In addition, Museum Victoria audience research has revealed that increasingly, a key feature of the museum experience is that visitors are looking for opportunities to express their personal opinions within an exhibition. Exhibitions in the twenty-first century are therefore interactive, in that visitors are now encouraged to comment on their experience. Therefore many exhibitions contain visitor's books or an online feedback opportunity, whereby museum visitors are able to contribute their individual comments and thoughts. While from one perspective the input may be feedback on the exhibition, even including additional information on objects within a collection, another aspect appears to be a greater need by visitors to contribute their thoughts which have been provoked by their exhibition experience. This is particularly true of exhibitions that stir up individual memories or emotions, as well as those that stimulate discussion and debate.

ETHICAL ISSUES RAISED BY THE DISPLAY OF MEDICAL COLLECTIONS

Precisely because of their confronting and controversial nature, medical collection displays can create moral dilemmas for museum curators. The primary ethical areas of concern in medical collection displays relate to issues of appropriate consent, and maintaining the difficult balance between avoiding harm to individuals or groups in any public display while also ensuring a benefit to the visitors in terms of the collection interpretation. It is important to recognise that medical exhibitions have the potential to exploit individuals, and can also either promote or destroy both professional and individual senses of respect and trust. These areas will be picked up and expanded more thoroughly in the remainder of this chapter, which comprises an exploration of the ethical issues specific to psychiatric collections, human remains, and collections of diversity and disability.

ETHICAL ISSUES SPECIFIC TO PSYCHIATRIC COLLECTIONS

Collections concerning psychiatry can be closed, private collections that were predominantly compiled by doctors and staff, or—far less common—psychiatric collections in public museums. These collections can comprise psychiatric hospital archives, photographs of psychiatric institutions, artefacts from a psychiatrist's office, or artworks and sculptures created by people with an experience of mental illness or trauma. These objects can tell many different stories that are medical, historical, institutional, political, and also personal.

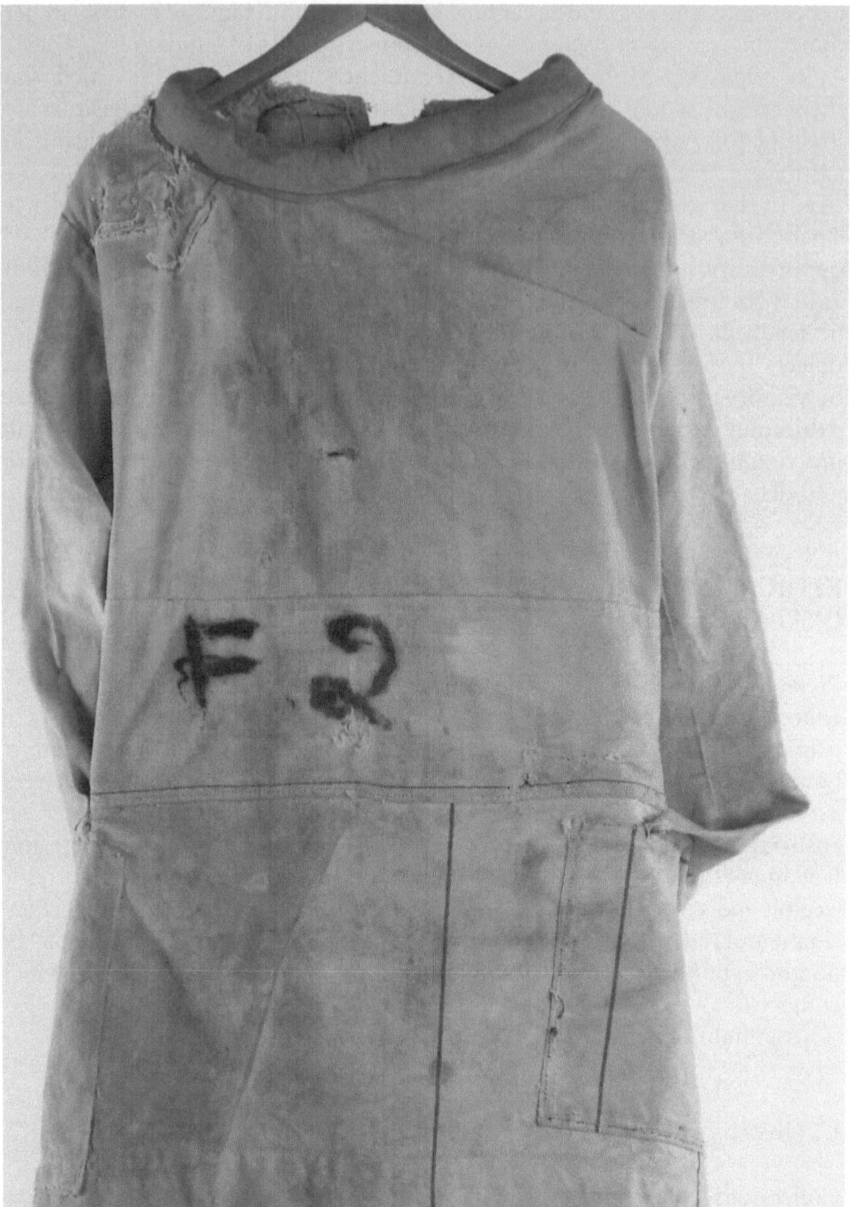

Figure 4.2 Straitjacket—Mayday Hills Psychiatric Hospital, Victoria, Australia, Cream Canvas, circa 1900.
Source: Photo by Jon Augier, Museum Victoria, Victoria, Australia.

The power in the display of psychiatric artefacts is their capacity to explore past medical practice, and to encourage public discussion and debate about certain historical and contemporary practices regarding psychiatric diagnosis, changing treatments, and the ongoing problematic issue of social stigma. Fundamentally there are three key ethical questions that curators need to investigate. Is there a bias in the story being presented? Can the curator ensure that any public benefit does not result in possible harm to an individual? Can the curator ensure that the displays demonstrate issues of respect, informed consent, avoid exploitation and ensure that issues of trust are maintained between the collector and individuals whose lives are being represented, and the visitors who experience the exhibition?

In presenting narratives of psychiatric history a curator must examine and determine whether one particular story is being emphasised at the expense of another. There is sometimes a tendency in museum displays to perpetuate the concept of past gruesome medical horrors in order to venerate the successes of modern psychiatric medicine, including the medical practitioners involved. These medical practitioners are often granted hero status, but in doing so many personal stories about individual patients and other staff are ignored.[4]

Consideration must also be given to how stories of mental illness and mental well being are told and displayed. How is mental illness being portrayed within an exhibition? Is it adhering to clichés and enforcing stigma? Is the display culturally representative, or is the exhibition exclusive rather than inclusive?

For example, one must consider the ethical display of artworks created by people who have experienced mental illness. Several questions underpin my own thinking about the display of these objects. Does such a display enhance our ability to empathise with those that have experience of mental illness? Should we display artworks that were created by patients, some of whom are unidentifiable, in psychiatric therapy programs, and should those artists we can identify be credited? Should artworks be displayed only with the artist's consent? What if the artist is no longer alive, or unable to provide informed consent? Who holds the power of interpreting the works and their 'meaning'? What motivates the visitors to view these artefacts and is it necessary to reveal an artist's medical history in order for their work to make sense? Is a display of therapeutic artworks potentially exploiting an artist and their life experience?

Interesting observations have been made about the Cunningham Dax Collection of artworks, which consists of over 12,000 historical and contemporary works created by people who have experienced mental illness or psychological trauma, collected since the 1950s. The collection is dedicated to the use of art in public mental health education, yet it carries the name of the psychiatrist who originally collected the works. It has been suggested that this collection has run the risk of appearing to be more about preserving and celebrating the work of a psychiatrist, Dr Eric Cunningham Dax, and less about the work of artists who have experienced mental illness and trauma.[5] The professional identity of Dr Dax has been enhanced by the collection that automatically links his name and personal history with the art he once collected and displayed to the public.[5] At the time of the original development of the Dax Collection, in the 1950s, the private views, identity and consent of the psychiatric patients were generally left unknown.[6] Since the 1950s the practices governing this collection have changed markedly, to the point where now considerable effort has been put in to identify individual patients whose work is contained in the collection, and attempts have been made to obtain consent from living patients to display their work.

It is also important to recognise that some medical artefacts in these collections, such as medical records, cannot be displayed because they contain private information about patients and staff, and are subject to State and Federal legislation in the form of the *Victorian Health Records Act* (2001) and the *Australian Federal Privacy Act* (1988). The restriction of access to such records, while rightly preserving the rights of vulnerable individuals, has from a curatorial perspective unfortunately overshadowed the experiences of psychiatric patients, and skewed the historical interpretation of events in psychiatric history. Rigid adherence to patient confidentiality has resulted in limited access to psychiatric medical records and difficulty in representing patient perspectives. These restrictions have led to a lack of historical research into the changes that have occurred in human psychology and psychiatry throughout the twentieth century.[7] Preserving patient confidentiality can also result in interpretive stories only being told about institutional events rather than personal stories of people and their individual experiences.[8]

THE ETHICAL ISSUES OF DISPLAYING ARTWORKS CREATED BY PEOPLE WITH EXPERIENCE OF MENTAL ILLNESS AND TRAUMA

Recent research has focused on examining the ethical issues associated with the display of artwork created by people with mental illness, in order to establish some guidelines to help inform curators and others about the sorts of issues that need to be considered.[9] The guidelines raise many issues that are critical when preparing to display any psychiatric collections.

People who experience mental illness are marginalised and stigmatised in society. Creative works produced by people with experience of mental illness can be used as a potent tool to challenge stereotypes. It is important to recognise that artworks are complex and can be interpreted from many different viewpoints: as works of art; as an historical artefact; as a record of art therapy; and as an expression of life experience.[10]

It has been proposed that the best way to look at this complexity of interpretation is to embrace the multidimensionality when displaying these works.[11] This involves drawing visitors' attention to the different dimensions of creative works by people with an experience of mental illness, including medical, aesthetic, historical, social, personal, and moral. In principle, each dimension is of equal significance and should ideally be integrated into a coherent conceptualisation. Although differences in context and curatorial aims will tend to emphasise some aspects over others, the visitor should be offered the freedom to decide which of these areas they wish to engage with. The rights and sensitivities of the creators of these art works must be considered paramount when displaying any examples of their work, and this may in turn limit the freedom of curator and audience to engage with these works.[12]

The research project *Framing Marginalised Art* (2010) established some broader ethical guidelines to be considered when showing such art works. These guidelines, which may be effectively applied to psychiatric collections, are intended to encourage curators to take on the difficult, yet important, job of exhibiting works created by people with experience of mental illness and/or trauma. Each institution will have different histories, resources, and aims, and will therefore need to adapt these guidelines to their own specific context.[13] In essence, the guidelines cover the following five key areas: embracing the multiple dimensions of the creative works; respecting the creators; negotiating ways to display work where it is not possible to obtain consent; respecting the audience; and building trust between individual artists, communities and the exhibiting institution.

Through a consideration of each of these areas briefly in turn, the full implications for ethical display become clearer. By embracing the multiple dimensions to the creative works, these displays should reflect their full richness. Where, however, the context or curatorial aims of a particular exhibition support one dimension more than others, the existence and relative importance of those other dimensions should be acknowledged in the exhibition. Through a process of respecting the creators of these objects, curators develop these exhibitions with consideration for and sensitivity towards people with experience of mental illness. At all times the artist's original intention for the creation of an art work—and the context in which that work was produced—must be taken into account when making decisions about how to display their work. Where possible, curators must seek consent for public display from the creators, because the artists' works may depict experiences that they consider private and wish to keep from the public gaze. It is also very important, where possible, to seek clarification from the creators regarding the form of any attribution of their works, as some creators may only offer consent on the condition that they remain anonymous.

The most difficult of these guidelines is displaying work where it is not possible to get consent. Curators might consider displaying works without the consent of the creator only when there is no other comparable example of work. The benefits of the exhibition, such as destigmitisation and public mental health education, must clearly outweigh any potential exploitation or harm to the creator of the artwork displayed. In these situations a curator must always protect the anonymity of the artist.

To respect the audience means that visitors must be given choice. Therefore the visitor should always be given sufficient warning about the challenging content of any exhibition, as they may find it confronting and disturbing. Where possible, curators should try to provide a safe and private space in which visitors can sit and reflect. Curators should not shy away from presenting material that might be uncomfortable, but they must clearly outline the rationale behind the exhibition, and take appropriate measures to ensure that all visitors are aware of what the exhibition contains. Given the multidimensionality of an exhibition's content, it is advisable to ensure that sufficient contextual information is provided and that it is both clear and accessible. In addition, it is important to supply leaflet information concerning mental health or other support group contact details, for visitors who may wish to privately access such assistance.

Finally, it is very important to develop trusting relationships between the museum community, the mental health community and the broader community at large. It is crucial to consult regularly with the creators of the artworks and with mental health advocacy groups. Curators might also consider bringing to the attention of visitors ethical issues and dilemmas associated with the development of an exhibition, and inform them of the legal and ethical responsibilities of the exhibiting institution. The establishment of an Ethics Committee, with whom curators could regularly consult when developing an exhibition, would also ensure that ethical guidelines were followed. The global move toward corporate sponsorship of exhibitions requires curators to be cautious when considering this type of financial backing. This is particularly the case where a possible perception of conflict of interest may arise. Curators should not be placed in a situation where they have eroded their institution's credibility because visitors feel that curatorial opinion has been bought by a corporation or lobby group.

ETHICAL ISSUES IN THE DISPLAY OF HUMAN REMAINS

Human remains represent an area of medical collections that has recently received much attention, particularly with regard to the ethics of obtaining specimens and ensuring their ethical display. How institutions go about obtaining and displaying these specimens affects an institution's good will and credibility. Furthermore, the display of human remains touches on many of the same ethical issues associated with displaying psychiatric collections.

Within a medical context, displays of human remains have traditionally encompassed anatomy and pathology displays. Displays include wet potted specimens of human organs and, more recently, specimens that have been preserved by a method called plastination. These displays may contrast healthy and diseased tissues. They have conventionally been used to teach human anatomy and physiology in closed collections, to health professionals within educational institutions such as universities. Recently, however, this situation has changed significantly, and some public museums may display anatomical exhibitions that specifically aim to educate young audiences and the general public. This can be seen in The Human Body exhibition at Melbourne Museum and the human anatomy display at The Exploratorium in San Francisco. Human remains can also be displayed in many other contexts, besides medicine, and they are used to tell specific historical stories, reflect different cultures, and illustrate themes from anthropology and sociology.

There are specific legal requirements for the display of human remains. For example, Museum Victoria's display of human tissue is governed by *The Human Tissue Act* (2006, Victoria) which permits the use of human cadavers for post-mortem examination, therapeutic purposes, medical education, and research.[14] Written consent is required from the person concerned, while they are alive, before their body can be used for these purposes. In Australia, displays of human anatomy can be exhibited at museums that target the general public as long as the obvious primary aim is that of medical education. Currently these exhibitions can only display organs and cannot feature intact preserved human cadavers. The display of these organs does not provide information about the donor. As I have discussed earlier in the chapter, there are also legislative requirements governing privacy that restrict the types of medical information that can be divulged about an artist, creator or contributor, in a museum exhibition.

Historically, human organs displayed in closed academic museums have appeared as depersonalised specimens. Rarely is any information provided about the person, except perhaps a reference to an illness, or to age and gender. Some museum curators have argued that depersonalisation is a negative practice. Depersonalisation has a tendency to divorce visitors from the profundity of what they are witnessing—a once living person, rather than a diseased organ. Other curators, however, recommend that distance is indeed required if we want to reach a wider audience without causing emotional distress. Out of respect for the next of kin, university anatomy departments actually request that anonymity of the donor be preserved when displaying human remains. Therefore anonymity and consent are important issues to be considered in the display of psychiatric collections, including the display of human remains. Respect and sensitivity are concerns in the display of psychiatric collections, as they also are for the display of human anatomy. Although no longer a human presence, sections of the cadaver still remind us that these once formed part of a whole person. Recognition of this results in our respect for that person and their memory and leads to respect for their remains. Therefore, it is important to always treat all human tissue with dignity and respect.[15]

We need to consider why there is such a compulsion by museums to display human remains. Why are models, photographs and illustrations not considered adequate for teaching anatomy and physiology? Quite simply, viewing the parts of a person who once lived does more than just communicate the exquisite complexity of physical structure and function. It immerses the visitor in an experience that occurs at a more profound psychological, philosophical and spiritual level. One hopes that this powerful reflective experience can occur in a morally safe and non-exploitative environment.

Unfortunately, we do see exhibitions of human anatomy that have fallen victim to sensationalism and exploitation. The most well known is the suite of Body World exhibitions developed by Gunther von Hagens. The development of the technique of plastination of human tissue, initially for the purposes of teaching and research, has culminated in the ability to produce whole plastinated human specimens. Many blockbuster exhibitions have been seen worldwide with entire cadavers, posed in a variety of ways—sitting, playing chess, using a mobile phone or simply dissected to reveal internal organs. Considerable public debate has ensued about the appropriateness of such exhibitions.[16]

As educational, scientific and clinical justifications are central to the ethical legitimacy of anatomical displays, one must question the intention behind creating works of art from cadavers, when the role of anatomical education is relegated to a secondary interest,[17] and the venture is entirely commercial. Some commentators argue that the specimens are used as a form of entertainment that demeans and exploits the human body.[18] The transformation of cadavers into art is seen as jeopardising human dignity. Hagens' need to present himself as the sole artist of the Body World exhibit in itself breaches the issue of human respect.[19] Where does the issue of informed consent sit within these exhibitions? Medical professionals have questioned the actual anatomical learning that is achieved by the public with such garishly posed specimens. The issues of exploitation, profiteering and self-aggrandisement raised by the Body World exhibits have great relevance to the major issues to be considered when displaying psychiatric collections.

Visitors have also questioned the educational value of, and the motive for, such sensationalised anatomical displays. Unlike public museum displays of human remains, research studies have found that visitors to exhibits such as Body World criticised these displays for not providing enough scientific information, and felt that the exhibits were primarily a business enterprise.[20]

This discussion raises the important role of the donor. Anatomical displays need to be more personalised, where due credence is given to donors without divulging too much private information.[21] Consideration must also be given to how an anatomical display might be viewed from the perspective of the next of kin, and what implications this may have for maintaining respect and trust.[22]

DIVERSITY AND DISABILITY COLLECTIONS

The ethical issues governing diversity and disability collections also relate to the display of psychiatric collections. Collections concerning diversity and disability are varied, and they encompass both physical and mental disabilities. They may concern objects that relate to medical research, diagnosis, and treatment. They also include items that act as aids for people who experience disability, and may be creative works. Artefacts may also reveal the stigma that can be associated with diversity and disability.

Exhibitions relating to stories of diversity and disability present some curators with what they consider to be insurmountable problems. Therefore exhibitions concerning diversity and disability have been sidestepped in the past by museums, as these cultural institutions were anxious not to be seen as presenting or supporting a freak show approach that might encourage voyeurism and disrespect, exploitation and sensationalism.[23]

A persistent dilemma for museums is how to ethically tell the difficult stories that may range from psychiatric institutional history, war injury and disability history, to personal experiences of pain and distress. In contextualising artefacts from these collections, should a link with a disability be made explicit when it might not otherwise be obvious to the visitor? How can the material be interpreted in ways that reflect and incorporate perspectives and insights from people who experience a disability?[24] By contesting reductive stereotypes, addressing difficult stories surrounding disability histories, and presenting the diversity of disability experiences, museums have the capacity to challenge our understanding of what disability has meant to society in the past, and what it could mean in the future.[25]

Curatorially, we need to consider the sorts of stories that we tell regarding diversity and disability. Traditionally, people with disability have been described as victims who suffer, when perhaps it is time to change that perspective and portray them as part of the rich diversity within human society. As curators we must ensure that we are dissipating and not enforcing the stigma of disability. A richer museum experience will be achieved by ensuring that stories are told from a personal perspective, and that the displays have been ethically developed with considerable consultation with individuals and communities.

CONCLUSIONS

Visitors expect contemporary museums to be visionary, and that museum professionals conduct themselves at the highest level of professional practice. Implicit in this is the expectation that museums are entirely ethical in their approach to the acquisition and display of psychiatric collections. This is particularly the case for museums that are financed, partially or in total, by government awarded tax-payer funds. In contrast, privately developed exhibitions, particularly those that are run as profit-making enterprises, have far less community pressure to conduct their business in a strictly ethical manner.

The confronting and controversial nature of exhibitions that feature medical collections seduce, connect, and captivate many of their visitors.

At the same time, they also have the capacity to alienate, revolt and distress the viewing public. Any exhibition of items from a medical collection creates moral dilemmas that need to be considered carefully on a collection-by-collection, and object-by-object, basis.

Whilst the museum curator may, at times, feel that the resolution of ethical issues associated with psychiatric collections is insurmountable, a conscious embracing of the complexity of these issues will yield a rich, authentic and emotionally engaging experience for the visitor. As much as possible, the primary factors to consider when displaying such artefacts are the importance of consultation and discussions with the broader community, and to be sensitive and respectful of the stories that are being told.

NOTES

1. Ken Arnold, "Time Heals: Making History in Medical Museums," in *Making Histories in Museums,*ed. Gaynor Kavanagh, Making Histories in Museums (London: Leicester University Press, 1996), 15–16. See also Peter Leiberich and others, "Body Worlds Exhibition–Visitor Attitudes and Emotions," *Annals of Anatomy* 188 (2006): 567–573.
2. Arnold, "Time Heals", 15–29.
3. Ibid.
4. Catharine Coleborne, "Remembering Psychiatry's Past: The Psychiatric Collection and its Display at Porirua Hospital Museum, New Zealand," *Journal of Material Culture* 8 (2003): 97–118.
5. Belinda Robson, "Preserving Psychiatry Through Art: Historical Perspectives on the Cunningham Dax Collection of Psychiatric Art," in*'Madness' in Australia: Histories, Heritage and the Asylum*, ed. Catharine Coleborne and Dolly MacKinnon (St Lucia: University of Queensland Press, 2003), 195–205. See also Catharine Coleborne, "Exhibiting 'Madness': Material Culture and the Asylum," *Health and History* 3, no. 2 (2001): 104–117.
6. Robson, "Preserving Psychiatry," 195–205.
7. Ann Westmore, "Reading Psychiatry's Archive: Academic Medicine and Psychiatric Medicine in Mid-Twentieth-Century Victoria," in Coleborne and MacKinnon, *'Madness' in Australia*, 207–216.
8. Coleborne, "Exhibiting 'Madness,' 104–117.
9. Karen Jones and others, *Framing Marginalised Art* (University of Melbourne: Custom Book Centre, 2010).
10. Ibid.
11. Ibid.
12. Ibid.
13. Ibid.
14. Parliament of Victoria, *Coroners and Human Tissue Acts (Amendment) Act 2006, Act No. 59/2006*, http://www.health.vic.gov.au/__data/assets/pdf_file/0003/323328/htact1982 _amendment2006.pdf.
15. Alastair Campbell, Grant Gillett, and Gareth Jones, *Medical Ethics*, 4th ed. (Oxford: Oxford University Press, 2005), 49–71.
16. Campbell, Gillett and Jones, *Medical Ethics*, 49–71.
17. D. Gareth Jones, "Anatomical Investigations and Their Ethical Dilemmas," *Clinical Anatomy* 20, no. 3 (2007): 338–343.

18. Jones, "Anatomical Investigations," 338–343; Lawrence Burns, "Gunther von Hagens' BODY WORLDS: Selling Beautiful Eduction," *The American Journal of Bioethics* 7, no. 4 (2007): 12–23.
19. Burns, "Gunther von Hagens'," 12–23.
20. Leiberich and others, "Body Worlds Exhibition," 567–573.
21. Burns, "Gunther von Hagens,'" 12–23.
22. Dirk Preuss, "Body Worlds: Looking Back and Looking Ahead," *Annals of Anatomy* 190, no. 1 (2008): 23–32.
23. Richard Sandell and others, "Beggars, Freaks and Heroes? Museum Collections and the Hidden History of Disability," *Museum Management and Curatorship* 20, no. 1 (2005): 5–9.
24. Ibid., 5–9.
25. Ibid.

Part II

Material Culture and Memories of Madness

5 'Always Distinguishable from Outsiders'

Materialising Cultures of Clothing from Psychiatric Institutions

Bronwyn Labrum

On the outskirts of Goulburn, in rural southern New South Wales, Australia, there is a museum in a former psychiatric institution containing a wide range of memorabilia. One particularly striking display in Kenmore Hospital features an isolation cell, where the most difficult patients would be confined. Through the peephole in the door, a mannequin wearing a straitjacket can just be seen. A similar display may be found in Porirua Hospital Museum, in the North Island of New Zealand, where there is a 'seclusion room'. That room is part of the former 'F' Block, a ward for disturbed female patients. It contains a single iron bedstead with bedding, toilet pans, and on the wall over the bed a canvas [strong] dress and jacket and some nightgowns are hung. These individual items of clothing stand out in the context of the rest of the museums' heterogeneous collections, which range from architectural remnants, furniture and crockery to the wide range of medical instruments used to treat patients. In the case of the seclusion room, it is clearly intended to be the main exhibit, and the poignant garments dominate the display, as a recent documentary about the asylum makes abundantly clear.[1] These two rooms and their contents, housed in different asylums in different countries, reinforce the infamous horrors and grimness of Victorian psychiatry. For many this is an era clearly marked off from the modern period of drug treatments and psychotherapy, and certainly set apart from the present era of deinstitutionalisation and community care.

Of all the items of clothing shown, the straitjacket epitomises the psychiatric institution, whether, as in these cases, tied on to a mannequin or hung in a former cell. As the reporter declared when a new exhibition opened in Museum London in Ontario in February 2009, 'Straitjackets and lobotomies usually come to mind at the mention of a mental asylum.'[2] Film, fiction and non-fiction perpetuate the popular stereotype. But so do many scholarly enterprises. For example, Lee-Ann Monk's absorbing study of Australian psychiatric workers, *Attending Madness*, features a straitjacket on its cover, even though the asylum attendants would not themselves have worn such a garment. Staff would have been all too familiar with the various techniques of wrestling struggling patient bodies into these garments. The image does symbolise starkly what many of the staff had to contend with. Indeed their own clothes, especially the cost of replacing them, became a point of disputation in attendants' negotiations with their employers.[3] The same straitjacket also represents Museum Victoria's psychiatric services collection on the 'Treasures' section of its website, celebrating the 150th anniversary of this Melbourne institution.[4] (The other objects featured are an ECT machine, a ceramic bowl stamped with 'Lunatic Asylum, Victoria' and a photograph of the Beechworth Asylum).[5] One of the expanding archive of 'cool things' on the website of the Kansas Historical Society is a small, female straitjacket from the Osawatomie State hospital, established in 1886, where such restraints were used through to the 1950s.[6]

Despite the ubiquity of straitjackets and psychiatric institutions' uniforms in the popular and academic imagination, the scholarly literature around 'seeing madness' still revolves around images or visual culture.[7] Scholars in this area note that 'underlying our understanding of the mentally ill is the continued presence in society of older images of the insane, images that overtly or covertly colour our concept and serve to categorise them upon first glance.'[8] These have emerged 'out from everyday perceptions, rather than taking our terms ex-cathedra from psychiatrists and other "certified experts" (pun intended) on what madness really means.'[9] In this chapter I examine the way that the ubiquitous straitjacket materializes how madness is 'seen' through objects and museum displays, rather than visual representations, and how it reinforces everyday perceptions of Victorian psychiatry and its custodial and often violent nature. I highlight the way that the wide range of institutional clothing in collections is neglected in favour of more conventional medical collections, including instruments and other tools of treatment, such as the ECT machines, architectural remnants, crockery (as noted above), and other similarly 'hard' items. This is the reverse of what applies to many historians interested in material culture and collections, who, it is claimed, have focused instead on 'cushions and curtains history', the '"soft", decorative and visible', stopping at 'the domestic doorstep'. They have neglected the '"hard" (but fragile) things and networks', including iron, steel and bullets.[10]

I also look further—behind and beyond the domestic doorstep of both the asylum and the museum—to see what other items of asylum clothing have been exhibited, drawing upon case studies of key Australian and New Zealand museums, both publically-funded and those run by volunteers. The daily life of patients and staff and the psychiatry practised in these institutions, including the clothing worn and used, formed part of an 'Australasian' world and these institutions exemplify those shared enterprises and institutional experiences.[11]

In examining these examples of the collection and subsequent use of strait-jackets and other, less familiar, items of clothing from psychiatric institutions I am interested in how they function as examples of the material culture of insanity, long after they were worn by patients and staff.[12] How do they constitute the experiences of life inside those institutions? What is their purpose and meaning? How do they provide evidence of the intended and unintended consequences of custodial control and treatment? What do they allow visitors in the present to forget as well as remember?[13] And finally, what kind of narratives do these clothes tell us that other examples of material culture, such as medical instruments or the built environment, do not?

PRODUCING FITNESS FOR PURPOSE THROUGH DRESS

Clothing loomed large in the world of the asylum—a uniform of dark, 'sexless' and hardwearing garments set alongside the military and nursing livery of the staff. It was as important as the worn and chipped crockery, the buildings in which patients spent so many hours, or the various medicines and treatments they experienced. Clothing was also critical for the attempt at effective management and control by staff, whose garments clearly suffered as much damage as did the patients'. The clothing was intended to serve the functions of the substantial institutions that developed over the nineteenth and early twentieth centuries. The Victorian institutions from which I draw my first example were part of a network of asylums that had developed after the colony gained autonomy from New South Wales in 1851. A new institution was built at Yarra Bend, near the state capital of Melbourne, and it received patients from the gaol. In 1867 two rural asylums at Ararat and Beechworth were established and by 1871 the Yarra Bend Asylum was officially opened; in the same year the Kew Metropolitan Asylum also began receiving patients in the vicinity of Melbourne.[14] The New South Wales institution in Goulburn was one outcome of problems with overcrowding, which were regularly put before the state government from the 1860s. The new asylum would ensure that families could be nearer to their members when they were receiving care. It was also close to the railway. The state government purchased the land in 1879 and approval for building was granted in 1893–1894.[15] In my third example, the asylum at Porirua in New Zealand was built on rural land some twenty kilometres from the capital city of Wellington, when the first two asylums in the region became overcrowded as the city grew and patients from elsewhere were transferred to them: first in the separate settlement of Karori outside the city, which then became incorporated as a city borough (1854–1873), and then at Mt View, in south Wellington (1873–1910). Like the institutions in Australia, the Porirua Asylum became a large village-like complex with thousands of patients and hundreds of staff.

So what did patients and staff wear while resident in these enormous complexes and what were the meanings of their garments?[16] After being committed to the asylum, individuals were bathed and men had their hair cut. They donned 'serviceable' clothing that 'provided adequate warmth.'[17] Although there was no intention to create a uniform, a standard dress evolved and is represented in the museums discussed here. Male patients wore singlets, shorts, nightshirts of 'blue, grey and red stripes', linen pyjama pants 'shaped like baggy Bermuda shorts', blue striped or pink checked galatea or flannel shirts, grey flannel jackets and trousers, trousers and coats made of moleskin fabric (heavy cotton fabric, sheared to create a short soft pile on one side), leather boots (without laces because patients removed them), overshoes, and hats. Female patients, who were a much smaller proportion of the population, wore calico combinations or pantaloons (crotchless), cotton petticoats, black stockings, dresses made from galatea fabric (strong, firm, heavy white cotton, often striped) that were 'shapeless, heavy, dark, unattractive', with 'dozens cut from the one pattern', flannel skirts, bonnets, and shawls in winter. Hemlines followed contemporary fashion. Female patients did not wear bras or corsets, men and children did not wear underpants. Patients were often too lightly clothed in winter and, although staff distributed flannels and jerseys, many did not wear enough clothes. It was only in the mid–1880s that some patients obtained a second set of clothing.

There are numerous contemporary comments about the threadbare and dowdy appearance of patients in their prison-like dress. A contemporary report from 1875 noted that '[t]here are few patients so far lost as not to be able to appreciate the distinction between the ordinary dress of civilians and that which is furnished to them on their admission. A consciousness of degradation owing to the change may exercise a prejudicial influence on many patients, and may obviate or retard their progress towards recovery.'[18] Wearing such garments, patients 'were always distinguishable from outsiders.'[19] Inmates often knew full well what was happening to them. Charles J., admitted to New Zealand's Auckland Asylum, proclaimed in 1890 that he was an 'inmate', not a 'patient'.[20] To add insult to injury, patients had no privacy. In 1897, Alice Schoch, the Official Visitor to the Porirua Asylum, 'respectfully' suggested that the female patients should be given dressing rooms for 'at present they have to undress in the corridors, which is unpleasant, and as the winter approaches, very cold'.[21]

The Auckland Lunatic Asylum exceeded 300 patients in the early 1880s and had nearly 1,000 patients by 1910. Its staff found that strong dresses (made of canvas, like straitjackets) prevented 'unnecessary waste of clothing.'[22] Victoria's asylums used canvas and leather locked gloves, padded caps for epileptic patients, locked straitjackets (with 'strong canvas sleeves sewn into large pockets'), webbed trousers ('strong piece of canvas sewn between the legs'), child-sized straitjackets, and strong dresses ('blue, very heavy cotton, lined and quilted').[23] Unsurprisingly, patients protested and attempted to subvert the rhythms of asylum life, especially through destroying their clothing, which took on even greater symbolic significance than it might on 'the outside'. Yet this action only confirmed their unfitness for 'normal life'. Significantly, one of the key symptoms of madness that led to many female admissions was dressing improperly or immodestly or appearing naked, underlining the highly gendered nature of the admission and diagnosis processes.

It is clear that staff had to deal with difficult patients in an era before drug treatment and run an economically efficient institution with barely adequate funding. In the twentieth century, psychiatric hospitals, as they were now called, remained the poor relations of the public health system in both countries.[24] Conservative approaches to spending and reform, and the impact of the Second World War meant that clothing, as well as bed linen, remained in short supply. Patients' appearance continued to be seen in uniform or corporate terms, and neglected as an integral aspect of the presentation of an autonomous, functioning self. In a novel departure, Mabel Howard, New Zealand's new female Minister of Health in 1947, took a personal interest in patients and their environments. At her behest, clothing became more varied. Female patients who were considered 'able to appreciate it' received underwear and for the first time menstruating women were able to have sanitary towels. Shortages continued through the 1950s. Clothing was still not routinely considered to be part of patient dignity and comfort, however. Sometimes when patients were undressed in the evening, their clothes were dropped in a heap in whatever state they were in, and then the same garments were put on again, perhaps in a different combination, in the morning. Shoes might be taken from the ward collection, rather than being individually fitted or 'owned', and used for different patients depending on who was resident that day. Only on new 'rehabilitation' measures was clothing individually fitted. In the 1960s and 1970s individual ward sisters could make a difference by insisting that patients had their own clothing with their own wardrobes to put them in and that they were treated more humanely.

Staff, in contrast, explicitly wore uniforms. Such large institutions had a range of staff, including warders or male attendants, nurses on female wards, maids and housemaids, and medical attendants. Male staff wore quasi-military uniforms, while female nursing staff initially wore a uniform instigated by Florence Nightingale: a combination of dress and pinafore, cap covering the hair, and a cape for street wear. Some had high stiff collars and white aprons buttoning on to 'baby bodices' and stiff turned back white cuffs. Their white caps were high and frilled round the front. Later they wore blue and white striped galatea. Over time uniforms became shorter for women and less formal for both sexes, although white uniforms, caps and capes remained for some time. From as early as the 1950s and by the 1980s there was a move to street clothes for nursing and ward staff, under a different model of care. These became items that were, like the corporate clothing of patients before the 1960s, easily identified and proved to be collectable, as we shall see.

Asylum dress performed a number of roles as it was put on patients or as staff embodied it. Not only did it provide—or attempt to provide—decorum and warmth, it also constructed the social, cultural, and racial identities of those wearing it. Whether through the starch or gleaming buttons and badges of the warders and nurses, and the white coats of the medical men, or the standard issue dress and trousers, but without underwear, this kind of clothing attempted to instil new habits of meekness, compliance, discipline, and dependability. While staff members were able to project authority and control, the dress of patients embodied less concern with issues of self-presentation, let alone respectability or dignity. Clothing actively produced distinctions and hierarchies, and fitness for purpose. Through these processes it became an indicator of status or lack of it, and of conformity with, or forced departure from, social and community norms. Dress was particularly important for female residents, because the institution was trying to instill or maintain a certain type of dependent femininity. In the process, staff attempted to control bodies as well as appearances. Dress was as fundamental to these institutions as the architecture, the interior space, the daily regimes, the meals, and the interactions with other patients and with staff. An intrinsic part of the disciplinary apparatus of asylums, dress was a literal materialisation of power relationships and subjectivities that such institutions attempted, not always successfully, to create.[25]

ISOLATION CELLS AND EMPTY WARDROBES

Private museums established and run by volunteers, often on the original site of the asylum, are the most common form of psychiatric displays, and have become more numerous in the wake of the de-institutionalisation of former psychiatric institutions in North America and the United Kingdom. My two examples at Goulburn and Porirua share many characteristics, including the way they display psychiatric clothing. Seen as a 'vital piece of Australian mental health history', the Friends of Kenmore Hospital (FKH) collection remains in its original site at the Walter Liberty designed asylum in Goulborne, which opened in 1895. It is empty and remarkably intact, although suffering demolition by neglect, as the buildings are visibly decaying. The FKH collection was inaugurated during the asylum's centenary. Memorabilia was displayed in one of the buildings at the celebrations and its popularity led to the proposal of a more permanent display.[26] This led to the opening of the Kenmore Hospital Museum in the former male Epileptic Ward, 'to better house and display the vast array of exhibits collected from across the site and through donations from numerous interested people.' The collection includes every imaginable salvageable item from the hospital and site and subsists on fundraising and some small grants.

The museum's website invites visitors to 'Step back into a 19th Century psychiatric asylum in the Kenmore Hospital museum. The Museum is located in a former ward and closely resembles how it was in 1895.'[27] Visitors arrive at the dramatic isolation cell with its peephole, after proceeding through several rooms including the featured stand-alone exhibition. It creates an aura of secrecy and dread, and reinforces the stereotypes about lunatics and confinement. No pictures are allowed and yet the door is adorned with coloured strips directing your eye to the hole. Despite the amateur presentation of the mannequin within, it is one of the lasting memories for the visitor and feels like the culmination of the entire display. Visitors the day I was there had no trouble finding the cell and spent a lot of time around it. In terms of fascination and 'aura', the cell matches the ward above, empty except for hard wire beds crammed together and lining each wall, entered by ascending narrow stairs. Most of the general exhibition rooms do not contain any garments, although there are (empty) wardrobes from the wards amongst the other collection items.

A number of reasons can be put forward for the absence of clothing. The first is that it may also be a function of literally what has survived, and given that there is neither ongoing secure funding nor professional standards of collecting, conservation or display, it is easier to deal with the more robust items such as parts of building, crockery, sturdy furniture, sporting trophies, photographs, visual archives, and mechanical therapy. The architecture of the site, given that the museum is literally part of it, dominates everything.

Another set of reasons relates to the predominant focus of the museum. The absences are, in one way, deliberate, because it is about the staff first and foremost. The museum, as Doris Kordes found as part of her fieldwork for a historical study of Kenmore Hospital, is a 'memorial site created by former nursing staff' and she concluded, as I found when visiting it, that it has a 'nostalgic and celebratory view of the asylum.'[28] The focus is resolutely on the buildings, the grounds, facilities and staff experiences, such as the extensive sporting memorabilia, competed for and won by staff, not patients. When Kordes joined the Friends as part of her fieldwork, three-quarters of the ninety-nine members were former nursing staff. When I took the tour during History Week in 2009, the guide was a former staff member and nearly half of the fifteen visitors in the group seemed to be either former staff or those related to them, according to conversations along the way. As the biggest employer in the town and an organisation that kept staff for many years, the hospital was a focus for them of nostalgia and comradeship, as well as negative memories.[29] This latter point also complicates the dominating idea in the scholarly as well as popular view that these large asylums were 'out of sight and out of mind'.[30] While entry and exit was controlled, and many myths abounded about psychiatric institutions, they were clearly part of the communities in which they were situated, both in terms of employment and links to the local economy and society, and also in terms of official visits and community relations. Generations of the same family often worked in the same institution.

The tour commentary focused on the architecture and staff experiences and memories. It also reinforced the theme of such museums and collections being about the distant past ('then'), quite separate from this day and age ('now'). When we went into one of the former wards and saw the wet cells, where dirty patients were hosed down, stark contrasts were drawn between the 'bad old days' of institutional psychiatry and the difficulties patients caused, compared with the improved practices of the present. At one point in the tour, there was an interesting but inconclusive exchange between the guide and visitors about the merits or otherwise of community care. The mundane and everyday was not emphasised as the stories and building we were shown were all about the worst, the exceptional, the particularly memorable, and all from the staff point of view.

The collection developed by the Friends of the Porirua Hospital Museum (FPHM), which is the only one in New Zealand, is very similar. Catharine Coleborne has written about it in some detail, principally in terms of the questions it raises about the experience of psychiatric institutions in the twentieth century, and the role of the museum and its collection in people's lives.[31] The Porirua Hospital Museum, like Kenmore, had its genesis in the institution's centenary in 1987. A part-time curator and volunteers initially ran the Museum.[32] This arrangement was formalised after Capital Coast Health, the government body responsible for the Porirua Hospital and campus, announced plans in 1997 to relinquish the Museum, which was part of its mandate. The Friends of the Porirua Museum was formed and the former F [female] Ward block in which the museum was housed gained registration as a Category One building by the New Zealand Historic Places Trust. Again, many of the Friends were former staff. After the Friends and the Porirua City Council commissioned a review of the future of the Museum in 2003, The Porirua Hospital Museum and Resource Centre Trust (PHMFRCT) was established in 2006 to ensure the preservation of the collection and the building in which it is housed.

As with the Kenmore Hospital collection, this collection and display can best, but not perjoratively, be described as an 'antiquarian' medical collection with the addition of exhibits from the asylum farm, some patient artwork, photographs of staff, and patient casebooks and other administrative documentation.[33] Casenotes from 1911 are on display in glass cabinets,[34] while the rest of the items are on open shelving on plinths, on the walls, and in other free spaces in the room. The wooden building is groaning with material arranged in a broadly chronological fashion.

Once again, the seclusion room has the few items of clothing on display in the entire Museum. It is also reached after proceeding through the general displays. It is a featured exhibit on the Museum's website, where, apart from a general view of the main exhibition room, the seclusion room is one of two exhibits—along with nineteenth-century medicine bottles—to have its own image.[35] Other highlights itemised are farm implements; a yoke to carry milk from the farm to the wards; an insulin treatment chart; ECT machines; keys; a morgue box, locked medication baskets, and the building itself.

The detailed description of the seclusion room continues to resonate, although on the website the straitjacket, strong dress and nightgowns are not the focus of the text. It is the architecture and the main piece of furniture which are described in some detail:

> Seclusion Room—used right up until the late 1960's [*sic*]. A shutter was placed over the window to prevent violent people from harming themselves. The mattress on the bed and blanket are made of heavy canvas to prevent them from being torn up.
>
> The door is very thick and heavy—there are marks in door [*sic*] where a bed end has been bashed against it. The light switch is outside the room. A peephole at the side of the room allowed the nurses to observe the person in the room even if they were standing directly in front of the door. The walls are filled with pumice to deaden noise and as a fire protection measure.[36]

The advocacy role of the PHMFRCT means that the horrors are emphasized, and as with the Kenmore Hospital Museum, the display is closely related to former staff's views and focuses on objects from their perspective. Once again the patients are subsumed within their environment and are curiously mute—despite references to 'deadening noise' and torn bedding. Except for the straitjacket, dress and nightgowns in the isolation cell, and the casebooks under glass, patients are notable by their absence, rather than their presence. It is the clothing that announces that they were once there. While further account is provided in the museum of everyday life at the asylum, principally through sports and the large asylum farm, these represent the exterior, rather than interior experiences, the ones that male patients were more likely to have enjoyed, than the female patients who were more often sequestered inside doing laundry or sewing. The assistance that women in particular received at the asylum, seeking respite from onerous housework, from childbearing and rearing, and through repeated committals, is not part of these stories.[37]

FILLING THE WARDROBE AND MATERIALISING MISERY

In marked contrast to the lack of clothing in the Kenmore and Porirua museums, garments from Victoria's asylums have always been prominently displayed, although the way they have been shown and interpreted has changed significantly over time. They were first displayed as part of a broader collection in The Charles Brothers Mental Health Museum, at the

Mental Health Library in the Office of Psychiatric Services in Parkville, Melbourne. The exhibition was used to teach students about the history of institutionalised mental health care in Victoria and aimed to show politicians 'what happens when public institutions are not properly resourced.'[38] As Coleborne recounts in her chapter, Dr Brothers was a member of the Victorian Mental Health Authority from 1952–1963, an organization which aimed to reform and improve the mental health system. He began collecting psychiatric artefacts, records, and photographs from cupboards and workshops around the sites, when many treatments and associated objects from Victorian times were still in use. The collection grew to over 700 items and centred on the period 1848–1950, especially from the late 1890s through to the 1940s. In 1994 Elizabeth Willis produced a publically available, detailed catalogue which includes twenty-five pages of garments in the section 'Clothing the Clients and Staff', and twenty pages of straitjackets, locked gloves and so forth, in a section on 'Treatments for Psychiatric Patients'.

Most of the clothing in the collection was from Kew Metropolitan Hospital. The patients' attire and staff uniforms had been worn, but the restraining clothing was apparently new and found in the stores at the hospital, which adds an interesting caution to the perception that strong clothing was used intensively.[39] Contemporary photographs from c.1961 provide the only evidence of how the Brothers collection was displayed.[40] In one room there were heavy closed cabinets, open shelving and glass display cabinets around the walls, with ECT machinery, equipment, utensils and other artefacts set out. An entire pharmacy from the Ararat Asylum was installed at one end. There were iron bedsteads, a hydrotherapy unit, and a heavy quilted blanket that could not be easily destroyed was draped over a fireplace surround. Open casebooks from 1906 onwards were displayed, complete with patient photographs attached to each entry.[41]

The shelves held folded items of clothing. The clothing was part of a general collection made in sewing rooms at the asylums, because of the lack of institutional budget to buy clothing. Asylums normally required female patients to (re)train in domesticity, compelling them to clean the institution, sew, manufacture clothing for themselves and other public institutions, and do the laundry of inmates and staff. All of this was done by hand, in primitive conditions, and on an industrial scale. In 1899, for example, thirty-two women did the weekly and daily wash at the Auckland Asylum, New Zealand, including blankets and quilts for over 400 people. If a patient was compliant, there was a progression from laundry work to needlework and knitting.[42] Embroidery done by patients as part of their recreation also featured in this display. Whole outfits were hung on rods imitating the human form along a central long plinth. The garments included a female attendant's uniform and hat, and a male attendant's uniform made of heavy-duty, long-wearing serge. A striped dress made of heavy material 'for the better patients', locked gloves, and a restraining jacket, with leather buckles to fasten up the front and sleeves sewn into pockets, completed the grouping. In 1965 an extension to the museum and library were completed. Contemporary photographs show that the central focus of the museum was now a featureless patient in a bed, surrounded by uniformed staff represented by fully dressed mannequins.

The Charles Brothers Museum focused on so much more than straitjackets, lobotomies and ECT, yet its intended purpose and context of advocacy for improved services emphasised staff rather more than patients, in a similar way to the volunteer museums. The patients were featureless when represented and not given form in whole outfits or even hanging garments. Yet the inclusion of folded garments and sewing must owe something to the curator, Mrs Roma Emmerson, whose role is little known, although she published research on it.[43] So here a relatively novel aspect was incorporated. The display utilised similar, if largely improvised, techniques as mainstream museums, at a time when none had the resources, aspirations and professional standards that we would expect today. Many public exhibitions in the 1950s and 1960s relating to daily life and domestic concerns, including significant displays of historical clothing, were curated by women, whether formally or in an honorary capacity.[44] This was different to the later interest in largely elite designer fashion, as opposed to 'costume', as clothing collections were often referred to. Fashion exhibitions have become a feature of museums from the 1980s.[45]

The Charles Brothers Museum closed in the mid 1980s and Museum Victoria (established in 1983) received most of the objects in 1987.[46] A report on the collection and possible exhibition storylines commissioned prior to acquisition notes that the collection represents the custodial orientation of psychiatric care up until the 1950s, before it changed to that of a 'therapeutic community':

> The overall picture of life in a mental hospital is a grim one. Patients were dressed in unattractive 'sexless' clothing, the food was unappetising, monotonous and vitamen [*sic*] deficient, and the sanitary conditions were appalling. The stench, apathy of the patients were all too apparent. Hospital staff worked under these terrible conditions, many of them were from undesirable backgrounds and . . . there was little or no formal training for psychiatric nuring [*sic*].[47]

The author realised, however, that this picture might be a little one-sided: 'Obviously there were many people involved with the care of the mentally ill patients who were kind and tried to improve the general lot of the patients, but under such terrible conditions it would have been very difficult.'[48] The report noted that 'Mental Health has had a chequered history in Victoria to say the least, the exhibits should not be displayed if at all possible as a "chamber of horrors", patients suffered terribly, and the hospitals were dreaded and awful establishments, however a well balanced, and socially historical perspective should be sought.' Although the collection was fully catalogued and parts of it were shown to interest groups and items loaned to other displays, it was not until the new Melbourne Museum opened in 2001 that items from the collection were exhibited.[49] They have since been used in a number of exhibitions, telling a range of stories about madness, asylums, and psychiatry over the last decade. Unlike the displays at Kenmore and Porirua, these items were framed within a general, rather than medical museum, one that invites visitors to 'Explore life in Victoria, from our natural environment to our culture and history.'[50]

Psychiatric clothing featured in the Australia Gallery, in the section within it entitled 'Melbourne: Stories from a City', which 'explores the history of Melbourne, its people, neighbourhoods, workplaces and cultures.'[51] In contrast to the volunteer museums, the items in this display were worn mostly by patients in the twentieth century: a child's navy wool cape probably worn in Kew cottages, 1940–60; a c.1950 child-sized white calico dress, with widely spaced, fine red vertical stripes; a c.1950 adult's maroon wool dress, with blue pocket; a pair of machine-knitted blue cotton women's stockings; a pair of finely woven, black woollen women's stockings, with numerous darns and seams; and a grey cotton bonnet from c.1950, but which 'looks Victorian', and a pair of white canvas boots.[52] Here the patients and their clothing are foregrounded to give visitors a broader sense of institutional experiences, and to show that children, as well as adults, lived in these institutions.

At the same time, older exhibition paradigms were reinforced. The now iconic straitjacket, c.1900, 'well worn and much mended' with 'F2' for female ward on the back, mentioned at the beginning of this chapter, is there (see Figure 4.2 in Nurin Veis' chapter), as are several items of staff clothing including a pair of crown epaulettes worn on male attendant uniforms and used at the Ararat Asylum, c.1873–1950; a male warder's cap in a French military style, 1940–49; a male warder's uniform, c.1909–1940; and a single white ankle length nurse's uniform, used c.1911–1950.[53] Other nineteenth-century objects, used well into the twentieth century, were shown temporarily in other parts of the museum. A wrist shackle was displayed in The Discovery Centre (research facility) and is discussed in Veis' chapter in this volume; a pair of cream coloured canvas boots (without the laces) in the 'Big Box' in the Children's Gallery; and the straitjacket was in the 150th anniversary show, Treasures of Museum Victoria, and the corresponding online exhibition. The website is designed so that the 'texture of daily life in an impoverished and overcrowded institution is evoked by well-worn domestic objects, battered metal chamber pots and standardised clothing.'[54]

In 2008 two of the Museum's key long-term exhibitions were refreshed and transformed, which provided an opportunity for new representations of psychiatric clothing. Melbourne: Stories from a City became The Melbourne Story and a new exhibition, Mind: Enter the Labyrinth, opened in the Mind & Body Gallery. In Melbourne Story psychiatric care features as a key storyline of the segment 'Nationhood and Identity', which focuses on the period 1900–1920, when Melbourne became the first capital of the newly federated nation of Australia. The key messages the curator wanted to convey was that 'residents of Kew Asylum did not share in the general well-being of the new nation'; 'many mental illnesses were not well understood, but doctors hoped that a quiet, ordered regime would help patients recover'; and 'the Asylum population included many people who did not have a psychiatric illness, but who were still deemed to be "insane"'.[55] Under the title of Out of Sight, Out of Mind: The Kew Asylum, the display makes the point that the largest public building in Melbourne in this period was an asylum, housing nearly 1,300 patients, rather than a hotel or even the state parliament. Showing a photograph of the extensive buildings around 1890, the interpretive panel states that:

> Mental illness was little understood and patients at Kew rarely saw a doctor. Although many patients were helped by enforced rest and a regular routine, others languished for decades behind the asylum walls.[56]

The segmental panel also features the stories of three patients admitted in 1907 and 1908, complete with their photographs. In an adjacent large case individual objects reinforce the second and third messages, most of which are not items of clothing, and includes a piece of brown carbolic soap (made from boiled down kitchen fat with caustic soda, with almost no lather) and a cutter. The custodial theme, however, is well represented in the few items related to clothing: a locked glove 'used to prevent patients scratching or otherwise damaging themselves. They were particularly used to prevent masturbation, which was listed as a cause of insanity as late as 1939.'[57] The canvas boots appear again. A mid-nineteenth-century flat iron and a washboard remind the visitor that 'Washing was done in large laundries. Clothes and soiled linen were rubbed with soap by hand, and then boiled up in huge coppers. It was heavy work lifting sheets and work clothes in and out of the hot water, and hanging them out to dry.' Finally a reproduction piece of fabric is 'Reminiscent of the coarse, utilitarian fabrics used for clothing at Kew'.

In contrast to the few garments used to tell a story of Melbourne institutional development, the exhibition devoted to the brain and psyche reframes psychiatric clothing in an innovative and evocative way. It is tempting to think that the interests and interventions of the lead curator Nurin Veis, the subject of another chapter in this volume, drove the narratives in this particular way. Mind: Enter the Labyrinth contains two historical sections that use clothing items from the Charles Brothers Collection. In a segment about the past, 'What have we learnt about the mind over time?', there is a timeline with an adjacent display of small portable 'mind objects of the past'. Of thirteen objects, one is worn: a wrist shackle used for restraining patients c.1848–1900. A graphic treatment with historical images of confined patients asks, 'How do we recognise mental illness?', noting that it does not necessarily conform to stereotypes and misconceptions associated with what used to be called 'insanity'. A large cupboard-like wooden structure, which is actually an isolation cell, stands nearby.

The segment entitled 'Past treatments for thinking disorders' comprises displays about the history of psychotropic drugs and psychosurgery and 'psychiatric institutions of the past' take their place. According to the thematic label, 'Many patients were institutionalised for life because they experienced an illness such as post-natal depression, schizophrenia, epilepsy, bipolar disorder and dementia. The 'asylums' were under-resourced, and conditions were crammed and spartan.'[58] An imaginative display of women's garments is in this latter part. They are totally encased and the visitor is forced to view them partially, through two apertures, focusing on the bottom half of the garments as they are hung inside the case in front of a large image of the exterior of a nineteenth-century asylum, also mostly obscured. The effect is of looking up into a wardrobe from below, yet it contains garments that once again distinguish patients from 'normal' people. These garments span the longest chronological span of the museums considered here. Hanging inside the case is an early twentieth-century dress with large checks of reinforced fabric, sewn this way so that it could not be torn by distressed patients; a striped c.1950 dress; a dark coloured restraint dress; and a red c.1980 nightdress. The distancing effect of the display technique is mitigated by an interactive feature placed below the group object label, inviting visitors to 'Touch the fabric to see what the clothing from old psychiatric institutions felt like.' The patients come to the fore, as do the ordinary experiences of the visitor, although the custodial element is clear. Visitors are able to imagine a range of stories and experiences, and perhaps the unintended consequences of asylum life, through the gaps in the case (wardrobe). The potential for new narratives about asylum life are clear through these delicately hung and suggestive garments and the conscious interpretation.

A case to the left reinforces familiar themes, however. This is devoted to items of bodily control, such as a restraining coat, c.1900, made of a double layer of hessian, whereby the 'patient's arms were pushed through holes in the inner layer, then covered and restrained by the outer layer'. There is a webbed petticoat, c.1910, 'used to restrict leg movement of agitated and violent patients', and a mid-nineteenth-century padded cap, worn to protect the heads of epileptic patients. Wrist shackles and locked gloves complete the materialisation of misery, which, because the hanging dresses are partly obscured, dominates the whole display. This case declares that asylums are part of the past, something that western societies have firmly rejected.

CONCLUSION

In 2007, 'Pete' posted online a fascinating and lengthy comment to the message boards of the BBC programme *Ouch! It's a disability thing!* He was in the women's section of a major store in London's Oxford St, 'and for a moment I thought I was in the laundry room story cupboard of an old large . . . Psychiatric hospital. And believe me it was an 'orrible thought!'[59] In the shop 'a couple of dress racks had grungy/shapeless and shockingly patterned, not to mention damn ugly clothing hanging from them.' He was taken back in time to an era when

> Female inmates no matter what age would have been forced into these 'boil wash, one-size-fits-all' uniforms with name labels sewn in. People rarely rocked the boat and complained of the shockingly drab and heavy costumes they were forced to wear. Institutionalisation ruled and extra meds were written up for those that 'questioned' too much . . .
>
> It really did for me hark back to the days of institutions kitting people out in recognisable uniforms for the purpose of stripping out individuality from people.

His comments, unlike the exhibitions I have discussed in this chapter, draw direct attention to the mundane and often unremarkable daily life for patients in psychiatric institutions, albeit for a later period than is usual for exhibitions of madness in museums. Whether professional, scholarly and well-funded, or volunteer-run on very limited funds, these exhibitions constitute the experiences of life inside those institutions in particular ways. Partly because of the history of the development of the individual collections—whether it is Charles Brothers or the FPHM gathering evidence to advocate for better organised and modern treatment, or former staff aiming to preserve their own past in the form of 'Australian mental health history'—patients are often secondary figures, and their material culture forms a subset of things displayed. The purpose and meaning of the displays relates to who developed them and what they want to show. With a focus on staff and how these institutions were run and functioned, the material traces of bureaucracy, buildings, labour, medical restraint, and sometimes extra-curricular activities like sport, are put on show. All of these themes and the style of presentation emphasise the intended consequences of custodial control and treatment. The straitjacket, of all items of clothing, along with locked gloves and wrist shackles—all enduring items from the high Victorian era—remain the most potent symbols of daily life, the icons of the collections, and the most frequently exhibited items. They are not always well contextualised.

The unintended consequences of custodial control and treatment, or the challenges and agency shown by patients (and staff) in the face of largely impersonal regimes, are absent and are much more difficult to put into material form, although the use of strong clothing is suggestive here. This lacuna allows visitors in the present to forget what more recent scholarship on families and asylums has shown: that some patients wanted to go to the asylum and that some families were happy to have them go there; and that many patients were in for short periods or moved in and out of the institution when they needed to. Asylums and their regimes were a more significant part of their communities than the clichéd phrase 'out of sight, out of mind' suggests. The exhibitionary techniques and choice of objects analysed here also allow visitors to put exhibitions of madness and psychiatry firmly into the distant past, rather than seeing the continuities with the recent past or indeed, with the present.

This is, of course, also a story of gender. Women were the minority of patients in the world of the colonial Victorian asylum, and the soft material world associated with them, beyond the straitjacket and lobotomy, is under-represented in display. The focus on 'hard things' and the lack of 'soft things' like clothing, although a part of every patient's experience, when farm work or harsh medical treatment and restraint might not have been, shapes the narratives in these displays in significant ways. Even the Melbourne Museum's wider and more imaginative display of clothing conforms to the conventions I have outlined because of the immediate exhibition context. How these objects are collected, remembered and interpreted in a range of institutions in former settler colonies helps to create new narratives for the deinstitutionalised present. In the process new materialisations of power and subjectivity are also made. The potential for clothing to tell new stories and represent power and subjectivity in different ways has only been partially realised. This is not to suggest that these exhibitions of madness are wrong or false, but to argue that they are a product of their time and place, like other museum materialisations, and that we need to understand their gaps and silences, as well as what is presented to us.

NOTES

1. Kathy Dudding, dir. *Asylum Pieces*, New Zealand, 2010. See also Catharine Coleborne, "Remembering Psychiatry's Past: The Psychiatric Collection and Its Display at Porirua Hospital Museum, New Zealand," *Journal of Material Culture* 8 (2003): 110–111.
2. Katherine Atkinson, "New Museum London Exhibit Pleads Asylum: 'Cultivating Care' Puts Mental Asylum Stereotypes to Rest," *The Gazette,* 4 February 2009, http://www.gazette. uwo.ca/article.cfm?section= Arts& articleID=2054 (accessed June 21, 2010).
3. Lee-Ann Monk, *Attending Madness: At Work in the Australian Colonial Asylum*, (Amsterdam: Rodopi, 2008), 125.
4. Museum of Victoria, Treasures Exhibition, "Pathways—Controversy", http://museumvictoria.com.au/treasures/path.aspx?path=4 (accessed June 22, 2010).
5. Museum of Victoria 'Treasures' Exhibition, 'Objects from the Department of Psychiatric Services', http://museumvictoria.com.au/treasures/details.aspx?img=2&Path=4&PID=20 (accessed 22 June, 2010).
6. Kansas State Historical Society, "Straitjacket", http://www.kshs.org/ cool3/straitjacket.htm (accessed June 21, 2010).
7. For example, the classic survey of images of the insane in fine arts, medical illustration, and in theories of physiognomy and expression is Sander L. Gilman, *Seeing the Insane* (New York: Wiley, 1982), iii. Simon Cross's new

study extends the focus to include 'historical and contemporary media ranging across single paintings, songs and photographs depicting insanity to the more familiar mass reproductions of madness in the tabloid press, television and via the Internet,' in *Mediating Madness: Mental Distress and Cultural Representation* (New York: Palgrave Macmillan, 2010), 3.

8. Cross, 3, citing Gilman, iii.
9. Cross, 3.
10. Frank Trentmann, "Materiality in the Future of History: Things, Practices, and Politics," *Journal of British Studies* 48 (2009): 286–287.
11. Catharine Coleborne, *Madness in the Family: Insanity and Institutions in the Australasian Colonial World, 1860–1914* (New York: Palgrave Macmillan, 2010), 21–23.
12. Useful primers on material culture and museums include Thomas J. Schlereth, *Cultural History and Material Culture: Everyday Life, Landscapes, Museums,* American Material Culture and Folklife (Charlottesville: University Press of Virginia, 1990), and *Museums in the Material World*, ed. Simon J. Knell, Leicester Readers in Museum Studies (London: Routledge, 2007). For Australasia, see Bronwyn Labrum, "Material Histories in Australia and New Zealand: Interweaving Distinct Material and Social Domains," *History Compass* 8 (2010): 805–816.
13. Susan A. Crane, ed., *Museums and Memory,* Cultural Sitings (Stanford: Stanford University Press, 2000). See also *The Politics of Display: Museums, Science, Culture*, ed. Sharon Macdonald, Heritage: Care–Preservation–Management (London: Routledge, 1998) for an essential discussion of the politics of exhibitionary selections, styles, and silences across a range of exhibition types; and Bronwyn Labrum and Conal McCarthy, "Museum Studies and Museums: Bringing Together Theory and Practice," *Te Ara Journal of Museums Aotearoa: Special Issue: Museum Studies in New Zealand* 30 (2005): 4–11.
14. Coleborne, *Madness in the Family*, 25.
15. Doris Kordes, "The Arts of Care in an Asylum and a Community 1925–2004: Kenmore Hospital, New South Wales and Canberra, the Australian Capital Territory," Unpublished PhD Thesis, Australian National University, 2009, 69. See also Coleborne, *Madness in the Family*, 32–33, 53.
16. This section draws upon Bronwyn Labrum, "Hand-Me-Downs and Respectability: Clothing and the Needy," in *Looking Flash: Clothing in Aotearoa/New Zealand,* ed. Bronwyn Labrum, Fiona McKergow and Stephanie Gibson (Auckland: Auckland University Press, 2007), 119–121, and Bronwyn Labrum, "The Social Significance of Institutional Dress in New Zealand," in *The Berg Encyclopaedia of World Dress and Fashion, Volume 7: Australia, New Zealand, and the Pacific Islands*, edited by Margaret Maynard (Oxford: Berg, 2010), 334. Other items from Victorian asylums are listed in the Museum Register, 13.009, Victorian Mental Health Library, Royal Melbourne Hospital Health Sciences Library, Melbourne.
17. R. M. Hunter, "Historical Notes on the Auckland Psychiatric Hospital," *The New Zealand Nursing Journal* (February 1957): 19.
18. "The Eighth Annual Report on the State of the Auckland Provincial Lunatic Asylum [New Zealand], 1874,"*Auckland Provincial Government Gazette,* Auckland, 1875, 208.
19. As M. A. Crowther notes of the British workhouse in *The Workhouse System 1834–1929: The History of an English Institution* (London: Methuen, 1983), 7.
20. Case 1637, Carrington Hospital, Auckland (YCAA) 1048/5, Archives New Zealand, Auckland Regional Office, 468.

21. Bronwyn Labrum, "The Boundaries of Femininity: Madness and Gender in New Zealand, 1870–1910," in *Women, Madness and the Law: A Feminist Reader*, ed. Wendy Chan, Dorothy E. Chunn and Robert Menzies (London: GlassHouse Press, 2005), 59–77, and Bronwyn Labrum, "A Woman's World in a Male Universe: Treatment and Rehabilitation at the Auckland Lunatic Asylum, 1870–1910," in *New Countries and Old Medicine: Proceedings of an International Conference on the History of Medicine and Health*, ed. Linda Bryder and Derek A. Dow (Auckland: Pyramid Press, 1995), 196–203.
22. Cited in Labrum, "A Woman's World," 200.
23. Descriptions from the Museum Register, 13.009, Victorian Mental Health Library, Melbourne.
24. This paragraph draws upon Kate Prebble, "Ordinary Men and Uncommon Women: A History of Psychiatric Nursing in New Zealand Public Mental Hospitals, 1939–1972," Unpublished PhD Thesis, University of Auckland, 100–102, 118.
25. Labrum, "The Social Significance of Institutional Dress," 334, 337.
26. The information in this and following paragraphs is from Kenmore Hospital Museum, "About the Museum", Kenmore Hospital Museum leaflet, 2009, in author's possession.
27. Kenmore Hospital Museum and Tours, http://www.visitnsw.com/town/Goulburn/Kenmore_Hospital_Museum_Exhibition_and_Tours/info.aspx (accessed June 23, 2010).
28. Kordes, 40–41.
29. Volunteers at the Western Australian Mental Health Museum also interpreted their collection through the prism of their own experiences as staff. See Catharine Coleborne, "Collecting 'Madness': Psychiatric Collections and the Museum in Victoria and Western Australia," in Coleborne and MacKinnon, *'Madness' in Australia*, 191.
30. The name of the official history of Porirua Asylum: Wendy Hunter Williams, *Out of Mind, Out of Sight: The Story of Porirua Hospital* (Porirua: The Hospital, 1987).
31. See Catharine Coleborne, "Remembering Psychiatry's Past," 97–118.
32. Information in this and the next two paragraphs are from Porirua Hospital Museum and Resource Centre Trust, http://www.poriruahospitalmuseum.org.nz/the-porirua-hospital-museum-and-resource-centre (accessed June 23, 2010); Coleborne, "Remembering Psychiatry's Past," 99–100, 109, and a personal visit.
33. Coleborne, "Remembering Psychiatry's Past," 99–100.
34. For more on these, see Marguerite Hill, "Madness in Early Twentieth-Century New Zealand: The Patient Case Records of Porirua Hospital, 1909–1915," Unpublished MA Thesis in Museum and Heritage Studies, Victoria University of Wellington, 2005.
35. Porirua Hospital Museum exhibits, http://www.poriruahospitalmuseum.org.nz/exhibits (accessed June 23, 2010).
36. Ibid.
37. Labrum, "The Boundaries of Femininity" and "A Woman's World."
38. Elizabeth Willis, *Behind Closed Doors: A Catalogue of Artefacts from Victorian Psychiatric Institutions Held at the Museum of Victoria* (Melbourne: Museum of Victoria, 1994), 9.
39. Listed in the Museum Register, 13.009, Victorian Mental Health Library, Royal Melbourne Hospital Health Sciences Library, Melbourne; Suzanne Hunt, "The Charles Brothers Mental Health Museum Collection Report," 1986, unpaginated, CM/087/21, CM-Research-Charles Brothers Mental Health Museum Collection (Psychiatric Services), Melbourne Museum Archives.

40. Information in this and the following paragraphs is from photographs 09.056.1–2, 'The Charles Brothers Mental Health Museum' and photographs 09.57–67, 'Items of Clothing and Views of the Interior of the Museum', Victorian Mental Health Library, which I am unable to reproduce here; CM/087/23–1, Collection Management-Research-Psychiatric Services History—Research Material, 8.
41. Willis notes that after 1906 patient photographs were often included, 25.
42. Labrum, "The Social Significance of Institutional Dress," 337.
43. J. Krupinski, A. McKenzie, and R. Banchera, *Psychiatric Research in Victoria, Special Publication No. 9* (Melbourne: Mental Health Research Institute, Health Commission of Victoria, 1981), 14.
44. Bronwyn Labrum, "The Female Past and Modernity: Displaying Women and Things in New Zealand Department Stores, Expositions and Museums, 1920s–1960s," in *Material Women 1750–1950: Consuming Desires and Collecting Practices*, ed. Maureen Daly Goggin and Beth Fowkes Tobin (Farnham: Ashgate, 2009), 315–340.
45. Amy de la Haye, "Introduction: Dress and Fashion in the Museum," in *The Berg Encyclopaedia of World Dress and Fashion, Volume 10: Global Perspectives,* ed. Joanne. B. Eicher (Oxford: Berg, 2010), 285–287.
46. The Museum has added to the collection with items from Caloola Training Centre (Sudbury) and Mayday Hills (Beechworth). Members of the Kew Cottages Historical Society conducted oral histories and current museum staff have undertaken further research on the collection. Willis, 10.
47. The quotations and information in this and the next paragraphs are from Hunt, 'The Charles Brothers Mental Health Museum Collection Report,' unpaginated.
48. Ibid.
49. Elizabeth Willis, the curator of the collection, made strenuous efforts to publicise it: parts of it were shown to the Health and Museums History Group in 1993, and in 1998–1999 items were loaned to an exhibition on Victorian Asylums at the Medical History Museum at Melbourne University.
50. Museum Victoria website, http://museumvictoria.com.au/ melbournemuseum/ (accessed June 21, 2010).
51. Museum Victoria, *Annual Report 2001–2002*, 22.
52. Information supplied by Dr Charlotte Smith.
53. These approximate dates for the clothing are taken from the most recent research being conducted into this collection as part of an ARC Linkage grant held by Dr Nurin Veis, Professor Elizabeth Malcolm and Dr Dolly MacKinnon, with research assistance by Dr Lee-Ann Monk.
54. Museum of Victoria, Treasures exhibition, 'Objects from the Department of Psychiatric Services', http://museumvictoria.com.au/treasures/details.aspx?img=2&Path=4&PID=20 (accessed June 22, 2010).
55. Out of Sight, Out of Mind, Melbourne Exhibition Story Proforma, 1, Museum Victoria.
56. Out of Sight, Out of Mind, segmental label, Melbourne Story, Museum Victoria.
57. All quotes in this paragraph come from the relevant object label in the exhibition.
58. Label text.
59. This and other quotations in the paragraph are from BBC, Ouch! Disability Message Boards, Old Psychiatric Hospital Clothing, http://www. bbc.co.uk/dna/mbouch/F2322273?thread= 3932070 (accessed January 16, 2009).

6 Snatches of Music, Flickering Images and the Smell of Leather

The Material Culture of Recreational Pastimes in Psychiatric Collections in Scotland and Australia

Dolly MacKinnon

Sound has not traditionally been an audible component of the display of psychiatric collections. Museum collections have been primarily understood to comprise the conspicuous arrangement of silent material culture that reflects and privileges the visual traces of past institutional life from the perspective of staff, and only very rarely from the experiences of patients. The act of collecting, however, has been more inclusive and sound artefacts—by this I mean objects, such as pianos and radios, which generate sound—as well as sports equipment that generated an interactive soundscape between players and spectators, have been selected and incorporated into collections. But often these items are simply ironically grouped as the now silent visual evidence of 'recreation'. Yet what these Bakelite radio sets, seventy-eight revolutions per minute records, pianola rolls, amplifiers, cinematographs and sound recording equipment actually represent is more than just visual reminders of the chronological history of technology and its adoption over time within the asylum; instead, these objects also remind us of the regulated soundscape of asylum life. Therefore, these sound artefacts can amplify for museum audiences one of the many aspects of a gendered landscape and life controlled by medical staff and experienced by patients and staff alike. Within the walls of the asylum, everyday recreational objects were adopted and adapted to assist the colonial medical project that attempted to contain, control and ultimately cure patients within the extraordinary world of the asylum. They also allow us to 'hear' aspects of the gendered sounds found in the outside world that were used as regulated forms of recreation within the soundscape of the twentieth-century mental hospital.

Inside the asylum, patients and staff lived within the confines of a gendered landscape and soundscape.[1] Even the provision of the official types of recreation was gendered, with sport for men and piano playing and hymn singing for women. Certain well-behaved male and female patients were selected to participate in gender specific and segregated activities (such as music, dances, cinema, radio and sport), and on some occasions suitable patients from both sexes were allowed to gather together and even, under strict supervision, to mix. The survival of records, radios and pianola rolls, as well as film projectors, is testament to that gendered soundscape of recreation. As my previous work has demonstrated, within the 'acoustomology of the asylum' sounds were categorised into binary oppositions of normal or abnormal, sane or insane, pious or pagan.[2] Therefore a consideration of the acoustic aspects of any material cultural artefacts moves any consideration of objects within psychiatric collections well beyond just the visual and tactile fields and into the sonic realm.[3] But the act of collecting this material culture also reflects inclusions and exclusions, as staff chose what was to be kept and what was to be destroyed. Those items used within institutions, however, both the included and excluded, do offer another narrative voice in the process of constructing new ways of creating psychiatric displays.

This chapter draws upon Jaques Attali's *Noise: The Political Economy of Music*, adapting his theorisation of communities that purposefully identify the boundaries of their auditory and musical worlds by isolating, categorising, and classifying sounds while rejecting noises. I analyse the complex place of the soundscape of recreation, through a focus on examples of surviving material culture, including items from Museum Victoria's Psychiatric Services Collection of over 1,646 objects (which also incorporates the Charles Brothers Collection); objects from three closed museums at the former asylums/psychiatric hospitals at Ipswich, Toowoomba and Goodna in Queensland, some of which were also used in the Museum of Brisbane exhibition, Remembering Goodna; and two photographic images of recreation from the Royal Edinburgh Asylum, held in the Clouston Papers in the Lothian Health Services Archive at Edinburgh University.[4] This chapter considers sound artefacts and recreational objects from these collections dating from the mid-nineteenth century through to the mid-twentieth century. The early recreational objects for Australia provide the auditory markers of the colonial project with its gendered template that proscribed the occupations of men and women, as well as a segregated and suitable physical and sonic landscape that might have elicited a cure for madness in suitable patients. This chapter then examines how the intersection between gender, recreation and the asylum soundscape demonstrates continuity and change over time by the specific material cultural objects from the nineteenth and twentieth centuries that have been kept in collections and also by those that were used in asylums, but no longer survive.

Cultural historians have begun to tune their ears to the sounds of the past, and turn their eyes to the potential of archives that may contain surviving information about those soundscapes. My own work on 'hearing madness' has demonstrated that the physical segregation of men and women was matched by a gendered cultural soundscape of inclusions and exclusions, diagnosis and treatment that involved analysing auditory and visual symptoms.[5] While landscapes automatically provide a visual plain, sound also has a terrain worth charting for historical purposes, and the sound artefacts of material culture represent another way of accessing that plain for objects in psychiatric collections.

Karen Harvey insists that 'history is impoverished without attention to material culture' and 'considering objects, often those found surrounding us in day-to-day life, as sources . . . can help historians develop new interpretations and new knowledge about the past.'[6] But how do everyday material objects from the outside world differ when they function as part of the colonial medical project of treating madness? The cultural values of the British Empire that championed an English speaking, white, patriarchal, Christian (predominantly Protestant), concert-viewing, record- and radio-listening, film-going, cricket, football and golf-playing, and spectator watching colonial worldview therefore filtered the recreation provided for diverse demographic populations of women, children and men. For example, the asylum regime even categorised the practice of religion as a form of recreational activity. There were only two officially sanctioned religions in nineteenth and early twentieth-century Australasian asylums: Protestant and Roman Catholic. World religions from outside of these denominations were considered inappropriate, culturally irrelevant to the colonial project, ungodly, and therefore resulted in significant omissions from the acknowledged official soundscape of the asylum. In cultural heritage sites across the British Empire the physical spaces used for religious services for Protestant and Catholic denominations survive either as chapels or churches, or as small wall cabinets in wards, but not the religious regalia and paraphernalia used for the practice of these rituals. No such official space or provision was made for other major world religions within the asylum. Yet an example of a Muslim patient in a Queensland asylum offers a telling example of the complex asylum soundscape that is not reflected in the surviving material culture of psychiatric collections. Ali B., a 'Mohamedan', who 'wears a white scull cap', was committed to the Ipswich Asylum, Queensland, between 1915 and 1939, and was provided with the opportunity to practice his religion. He made and sold rope work to earn money, possibly so he could observe a Halal diet.[7] His casebook entries attributed this special provision to the fact that he 'can talk to the [Medical] Supt. about various places in India.'[8] Yet there are no artefacts in the psychiatric collections for Victoria and Queensland that actually reflect the religious diversity of the demography of the asylum life.

The cultural diversity of the asylum population and the many languages other than English that were spoken within the walls of asylums across the British Empire is rarely reflected in the survival of select recreational material culture that is collected. The exceptions are some wooden sculptures and drawings that have inscriptions in Romanian, and are held in the Museum Victoria collection. These art works were created by Stefan Baiesanu.[9] Baiesanu was 'born in Romania on 14th December 1913 . . . [and]

had been trained under "a famous French sculptor"' before being admitted to Beechworth as a patient in 1954, and dying at Royal Park in 1980.[10]

Within museums, therefore, any attempt to re-activate sound-based material culture by re-animating them and hearing part of the soundscape they articulate is a powerful example of Pierre Nora's 'tradition as memory that has become historically aware.'[11] In most psychiatric collections, recreational activities are represented by former staff who ventriloquise their own experience through those lives of the select patients they remember, the specific material culture objects they preserve, and the aspects of the landscapes of that institutional past they recollect. In her chapter for this volume, Barbara Brookes' analysis of the multiple and shifting functions of photography in both the working life of the asylum and in the ways photography is now used to remember the asylum demonstrates this poignantly. Here, I ask readers to see and hear how the former medical, nursing, and general staff who actively collected and are the custodians of their memories through the act of collecting have included evidence of aspects from that soundscape. By tuning our ears to the gendered nature of those sounds we can offer a new aspect and sensory dimension to the practice of displaying madness. The views of former staff remain conspicuous by their selection, construction and interpretation of their psychiatric collections, while the multitudes of patients in their charge either murmur at us or remain mute. Shifts in focus and new directions in psychiatric memorials and interpretations have begun to redress this patient absence, as Nathan Flis and David Wright's chapter demonstrates for the Canadian context, and as the patient audio features discussed by Jo Besley and Mark Finnane in their chapter about the Museum of Brisbane public exhibition Remembering Goodna articulate. Yet sound still remains in its infancy as a mechanism for display in the area of psychiatric collections.

RECREATIONAL SOUNDSCAPES

Using examples of recreational images and objects taken from psychiatric collections in Australia and Scotland, I consider how these collections reflect evidence of official gendered recreation. I also examine how these collections largely reflect the recreational experiences of men rather than women. Building on my earlier work, I show how our histories of psychiatry can be enriched by analysing sound, and that the asylum is a place where we can recover evidence of those medical and gendered sounds and filters that articulate perceptions of madness and normality.[12] For the purposes of this chapter, I focus on the sounds of gendered recreation, which the medical authorities understood to include also select forms of religious worship. The inclusions and exclusions of recreational material culture, including sound artefacts from psychiatric collections, call out for our attention, should we tune our ears towards the gendered colonial and post-colonial medical environment that they represent.

Evidence of both official and unofficial recreational activities exists in the material culture of psychiatric collections, as well as through objects I have viewed on site visits to former psychiatric facilities at Goodna, Ipswich and Toowoomba in Queensland, which have not made it into these collections and exhibitions largely because of their size, and/or because they are considered everyday sorts of items. For example, on a visit to the Challinor Disability Centre after its closure in 1998, an upright piano remained in the recreation hall, and on the recreation hall floor were loose scattered pages from Ira D. Sankey's compilation *Sacred Songs & Solo* that was republished from the late nineteenth century onwards.[13] Only the four music stands from this recreation hall survive in a private collection. In another part of the Ipswich complex a dilapidated upright piano stood in a former ward on a urine-soaked carpet in a derelict ward marked for demolition. Traces of the male sports fields (that catered for golf, football and cricket), the oversized garden dominoes board in the male ward airing-yard, and male tennis courts, however, did survive and some were adapted for reuse, and subjected to a lavish and costly makeover as part of the new Ipswich Campus of The University of Queensland from 1999.

Recreational spaces within the asylum in Australia, New Zealand, Scotland, and North America were purpose-built spaces. Sometimes, however, the pressure on space within the asylum was so great that even the recreation hall was requisitioned for use as a storeroom or dormitory. Recreational activities also could be held for short periods of time each day, each week, during the summer or winter months or annually in wards and airing yards or sports fields. Many of these recreational spaces have, with the decommissioning of psychiatric sites across the globe, either been demolished or adapted for reuse as residential complexes or university campuses. Yet the recreational soundscape of the asylum that is reflected in surviving sound artefacts from official recreational activities is testament to the contested space where some but not all patients were allowed to contribute. Equally, the exclusion, muffling or silencing of the majority of patients also speaks volumes about the soundscape of everyday life, and the intentions of the colonising medical project to civilise, instill appropriate gender behaviour, and normalise patients within the asylum. As I have demonstrated, the asylum ball, an iconic feature of asylum history, was both a visual and auditory advertisement for the successes of the colonial medical project in the treatment of madness, but it achieved this by creating a highly selective, restricted and gendered soundscape comprised of a limited number of suitable patients accompanied by asylum staff.[14] By adapting Attali's model of the political economy of noise for an asylum, the sounds, noises and silences that are generated by the material culture of recreation that survives reflects how religious services resonated sounds of religious conformity and the colonial push for Christianity, and how gender distinctions were made audible through the different forms of recreation.

In the nineteenth and twentieth centuries the asylum implemented a 'sonic straitjacket' in which one particular cultural view then proscribed a gendered and class-based interpretation of acceptable speech, silence, dress, movement, and recreation.[15] The regulation of the official recreation and sport provided within asylums demonstrates ample evidence of this practice, and the cultural specificity of sporting activities deployed across the asylums of the British Empire has yet to be fully researched. Furthermore the archival, photographic and material culture found in psychiatric collections contains mute images and accounts of sporting activities such as cricket, football, tennis, curling, and golf, used as official recreational pastimes in the asylum. Yet remarkably few of these sporting objects survive in psychiatric museum collections precisely because they were useful everyday items that, although used within a medicalised environment, had uses beyond the asylum. Among the items in the Museum Victoria collection, for example, is an extremely rare survival of a cloth ball which was 'found under floorboards of one of the oldest buildings (1880s) at Caloola Training Centre,' which was the former nineteenth-century Sunbury Asylum in Victoria.[16] From the late 1870s onwards certain male patients were employed in workshops in asylums that produced items of clothing and boots, 'cricket and foot balls'.[17] So rather than the material objects themselves, what then remains in these collections are the images of the men and women at asylum balls, sporting carnivals, and male sports teams, along with any trophies these male teams won—noisy activities often only captured within a single photographic frame as a hushed static image. Yet while trophies have also been seen, erroneously, to represent only staff recreation and sporting achievements, it is clear from the survival of a 'shield' for the 'Mental Hospital Patients Cricket Association'—which lists the 'names of the winning teams for each year between 1957 and 1964–1965'—that patients did participate in sporting competitions and fixtures at Ararat in Victoria.[18] A similar trophy survives for 'Mental Hospital Patients Football Association' for 1964–1965 for Sunbury Mental Hospital.[19] While staff have collected these items, one wonders what former patients would have selected or rejected as items they wished to display. As Fiona R. Parrott's chapter demonstrates, for the twenty-first century, individual men and women who were patients revealed very strong and clear views about why they chose to decorate, or chose not to decorate, their rooms in locked wards. These patients' voices also need to be added to the contextual narratives to inform both the former staff who collected psychiatric objects and also the museum staff who make this material accessible to a wider public through the act of physical or online display.

Furthermore, a consideration of the provision of sporting recreation in Australia and Scotland demonstrates that the practice was not uniform across the British Empire, with the sports offered being partly determined by climate and cultural preference. In Scotland during the mid-nineteenth century, the *Morningside Mirror*—the newspaper of the Royal Edinburgh Asylum—told its readers beyond its walls in the winter of 1865 that 'cricket has in the meantime been suspended, partly owing to the depth of snow, and partly to the evenings being so short.'[20] The survival of a single late nineteenth-century sepia photograph of select male patients and staff from the Royal Edinburgh Asylum involved in *bonspiel* or curling on a frozen lake is testimony to the types of initiatives asylum staff took in providing outdoor amusements that incorporated local sports.[21] Edinburgh in the winter offered staff limited daylight for outdoor activities for the public and private patients at the Royal Edinburgh Asylum. Unlike the summer months, when the sun rose early in the morning and the gloaming stretched beyond 10 p.m. each night, in winter daylight appeared by mid-morning and darkness arrived in the mid-afternoon. To combat the shortness of the day, staff and patients played on into the darkness by the light of bonfires and torches. The initiative taken by staff in 1865 that 'curling is being tried instead [of cricket], and [that it] succeeds capitally' demonstrates the adaptability of recreation to suit the climate, interests and inclinations of asylum staff and select patients.[22] The regular winter reports of the REA Curling Club that appear in the asylum newspaper, *Morningside Mirror,* indicates how psychiatric collections of archives and photography can recover glimpses of select recreational experiences (and if ever released and published in public, display and promote the asylum in a good light). Given the prevalence in the twenty-first century of nations who sent teams to the curling competition at the Canadian Winter Olympics in 2010, this Scottish example of a late nineteenth-century asylum curling club suggests that further evidence of this recreational practice may well be found in European and North American asylums should we care to look for them. Behind the still, silent image of men intent on playing their game, the sounds of the swishing of brushes on the ice, and the cheer that goes up with the click of one of the granite curling stones hitting another, is tantalisingly beyond the grasp of the medium that records this event. The curling equipment, which is valuable and useful beyond the asylum, is also no longer extant and is only preserved within a single photographic image, as well as in the regular accounts of the ongoing success of the Asylum curling club in the Asylum newspaper.

The everyday recreational items from the outside world when they are found within the closed world of the asylum are evidence of a controlled, contained and restrictive environment of official recreation within a medicalised environment and soundscape. These everyday items, when they are selected by staff for commemoration and then are displayed within a museum collection, do not represent the ready availability of recreation in the everyday lives of all patients, but rather a gendered and select regime available to only a few of the patients and staff. Given this, can the agency

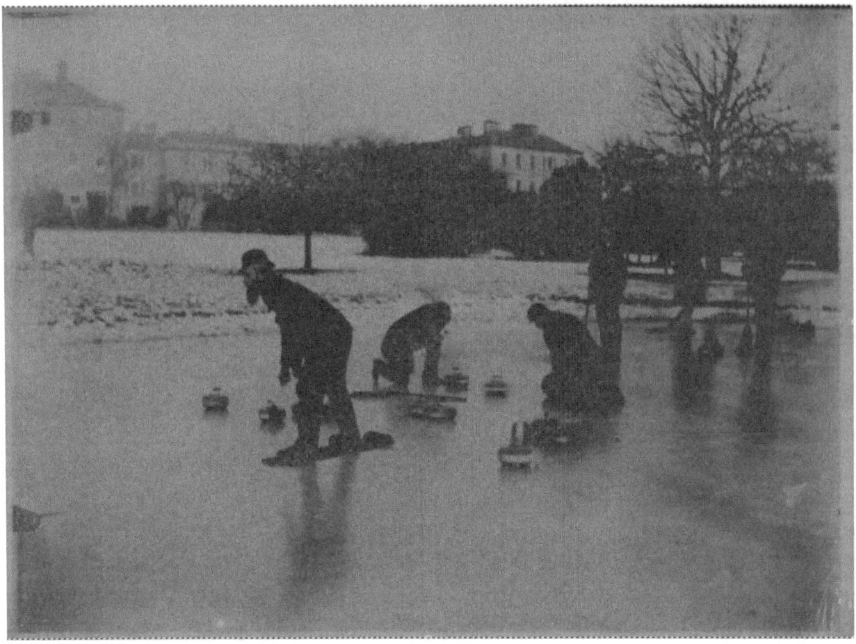

Figure 6.1 Staff and patients curling, Royal Edinburgh Asylum, Scotland, c. 1880s. *Source*: Record Ref: GD16, Box 3 and reproduced by permission of the Lothian Health Services Archive, Edinburgh University Library.

of patients ever be reclaimed when examining the soundscape generated by certain material objects? From the perspective of museum display, how has sound been utilized, what gendered material culture sound artefacts have been retained and which have been omitted from collections?

HEARING PSYCHIATRIC COLLECTIONS

The potential sounds of music from within a glass case are not the things we might expect from psychiatric collections. Sounds and noises are something we instinctively associate with institutions dealing with mental illness, but not so the strains of music, both live and pre-recorded. Such ordered sounds are less obviously associated with these places. Yet music holds a therapeutic value that has a long and distinguished history.[23] Equally, radio broadcasts that were played into the gender segregated asylum wards through a centralised radio system linked the outside world to the inside world through the filtered control of the staff. Asylums were filled with sounds.

Museums around the globe have readily used sound in their general exhibitions by either commissioning the composition of ambient soundscapes intended to evoke a sense of space, place and culture, or by reactivating sound-based material culture (records, audiotapes, film, television or videos). Today, in many historic buildings and museum galleries, sound loops containing voiceover narratives accompanied by soundscapes of street noises or site-specific ambient sounds intended to recreate the auditory feel for the past, automatically accompany exhibits, and activate as visitors enter each space. An alternative to this collective soundscape is the individual audio tour. Here the tourist is nestled into a personalised journey, which they can control by activating, stopping, skipping or replaying the audio tour. The narrator's lips speak words directly into the listener's ears. The only thing missing is the feel of the speaker's warm breath. The headphones of the individual audio tour act as baffles shielding the listener from the unwanted soundscape of twenty-first century reality. The sounds of historical authenticity require a closed soundstage.

Mary Hutchison and Lea Collins' recent work on three museum sound installations was informed by James Clifford's focus on 'the interaction of colonial encounters and how the inequalities of these may be turned around through exhibition practices that start with the agency of those whose material had been collected as part of the colonial enterprise.' [24] Hutchinson and Collins' approach provides a useful parallel comparative trajectory here for psychiatric collections.[25] Also, with the focus of this chapter being on psychiatric collections, I am excluding the commercial sound and light 'tourist ventures' that play on the fear of the ghosts of former mental institutions.[26]

The world of museology has also begun to address the role of audio interpretations in their displays. Most often individual audio guides are used for special feature touring exhibitions, where the headphones cocoon the listener into an instructive, interpretative, exclusive soundscape with voiceover—sometimes with background sounds along with any music, to create a sense of time and place. As Hutchison and Collins observe, 'typically audio representation in museums is most concerned with personal story as historical experience, while public art sound installations work with voices and sounds to create a sense of place. Again typically, the former is associated with the instructional intentions of museums, the latter with imaginative interpretation.'[27]

Within the area of psychiatric collections, Museum Victoria in their permanent display—The Mind and Body Gallery: Enter the Labyrinth, curated by Dr Nurin Veis—includes a section on mental health and provides examples of psychiatric conditions and personal experiences recounted on film by actors, while the Museum of Brisbane (MOB) exhibition, Remembering Goodna, utilised sound files of personal stories and experiences through headphones. Here the archetypal mythology of the asylum as silent, and the anonymity of the majority of faceless and voiceless patients, has been replaced by representations of the individual voices of personal patient experience.

SOUND ARTEFACTS AS INCLUSIONS AND EXCLUSIONS

But some sound artefacts that constitute large physical objects, such as grand pianos and upright pianos, or cinematograph machines, are less easily accommodated in psychiatric collections or in public displays. While they have remained *in situ* in recreation halls and wards as these institutions were scaled down and eventually closed over time, they have not been incorporated into psychiatric collections. Take for example the 1878 Steinway & Sons grand piano that in 1997 remained at Baillie Henderson hospital in Toowoomba and was used in the asylum Recreation Hall. Elsewhere I suggest that 'It stands silenced and abandoned, no longer a medical vehicle for recreation, but now transformed into a silent medical memorial.'[28] But inscribed on this instrument is the graffiti of former unknown patients, and 'the black lacquered surfaces [have] fulfilled an unforeseen function.'[29] While sport was the domain of men, the piano was considered the domain of women, the home, and 'domestic medicine.'[30] Carved into the piano's many surfaces are 'initials (some of which are illegible) and pictures', including in capitals '"JACKIE STEAVE" [then scratched out], "Margaret Jack", and in cursive script "Tracey"'.[31] This piano offers a range of official and unofficial examples of recreational activities, and forms the medium onto which medical views and some female patient responses are simultaneously inscribed.

Sound artefacts stand inert and mute before us, only taking on their full significance when, where possible, they can be reactivated and their context fully understood. There was a proliferation of printed music, musical instruments, and musical technologies (gramophones and radios) in the twentieth-century mental hospitals in the British Empire. For example, in the 1918 Annual Report for Goodna Mental Hospital, Queensland, 'musical instruments, either pianos or gramophones, are now supplied to all wards.'[32] By the early 1930s wireless radio was installed in Australian general and mental hospitals. In 1931 the Ipswich Mental Hospital in Queensland 'chiefly raised [funds] through the voluntary efforts of staff and their friends' to install a wireless system, which brought music and news of state and national sports into the gendered asylum wards. Some of the patients expressed their willingness to subscribe a few shillings towards this fund, which was also the case regarding the installation costs of over £447 at Goodna Hospital, Queensland, in 1935. There is a 'large, dark brown, oval shaped Bakelite electric radio' with 'two missing control knobs, one for volume and one for station selection' held in the Museum Victoria collection.[33] Were these control knobs removed by a member of staff to proscribe the soundscape contents and volume for the ward, or have the controls been removed by a patient demonstrating their individuality, agency and ability to impose their choice on the ward soundscape? The crackle and static of the central radio, kicking into life across the hospital ward, allowed for brief periods of time the musical and sporting sounds of the outside world inside the restricted and medicalised world of the psychiatric hospital.[34] Here is Attali's political economy of noise—where sound takes on loaded meanings, multiple values, and is an audible representation of asylum regulation and control.

The practice of collecting, therefore, often results in an incomplete and gendered picture of asylum life with a heavy leaning towards medicine, medical men, male staff, and (to a far lesser extent) male patients, and collections in which female staff, and especially female patients, are under-represented. Furthermore, psychiatric collections are traditionally seen and not heard which again limits the potential of their content.

THE STRAINS OF FEMALE RECREATION

When material culture is the focus, regardless of whether objects have been included or excluded from a collection, then the gender imbalance and full assortment of the everyday sound objects available in the material culture of the asylum can be rediscovered. Imagine, for example, in the early twentieth century, during the height of summer, a female patient's hands spring nimbly across the upright piano keyboard, deftly accompanying the flickering images of the silent film projected onto the large screen in the darkened and crowded recreation hall at the Ipswich Asylum, Queensland. The hall is filled with segregated male and female patients and staff who make their own contributions to this ambient soundscape.[35] From 1929 onwards, week after week, Amy M. follows this ritual, and 'frequently plays piano at the pictures.'[36] But over a four-year period her casebook entry records that the quality of her accompaniment has begun to diminish, and by 1933 'she cannot play very accurately now.'[37] Equally, her medical state was described by the visual and auditory observations of the medical men compiling her case notes, for they saw and heard that Amy M. was 'quiet and well behaved. Sews in [the] workroom.'[38] Amy was one of many female patients and female staff who provided the free piano accompaniment to the silent films in Australian asylums.

From 1910 onwards, film (while subjected to censorship) in Australian asylums was considered beneficial for patients, as they created an interactive and realistic link to the outside world. Hollywood silent films were played with live piano accompaniment. The installation of cinematographs in Australian institutions after World War I meant that films could be easily shown, and that the capital investment in this new technology was justifiable because of the benefits to certain patients. The only silent film that we know was shown in an Australian asylum is Roscoe 'Fatty' Arbuckle's *The Butcher Boy* (1917), which also starred Buster Keaton. After the invention of 'talkies' with an inbuilt soundtrack, there was no longer a need for either a staff member or patient to provide live piano accompaniment. Philanthropy also saw the latest technologies brought into the asylum and the

Herald newspaper in Melbourne, Victoria, presented Mont Park Hospital with a Krupp film projector complete with Cinesound enabling them to show, each Friday night, 'talkies.' Thus, the more intimate accompaniment provided at Ipswich Asylum by patient Amy M., which demonstrated a personal connection between moving images and live piano accompaniment, was replaced by soundtracks. Amy's practice of selecting musical snatches from the commercially produced thematic piano volumes, or studio music crib sheets—comprising pre-selected themes from classical music to accompany and mark the changing moods of the film's scenes—established for audiences the intended emotional connections between the sounds they heard and the images they saw, was replaced by a pre-recorded musical sound score. Whether the music was provided live by an accompanist or provided by a sound track, film music became a template for the dissemination of the twentieth-century stereotypical connections of mood with music. Yet the additional sounds generated from within psychiatric facilities during these film shows are much harder to recreate. For while the spaces in which these recreational activities were performed do survive—even the recordings that were played survive—we cannot recreate the dampening effects of and sounds from the bodies of the staff and patients who attended these musical events. Very rarely are the individual experiences of patients, and especially women such as Amy M., recorded.

GENDERING RECREATION

Yet the silent surviving pianola rolls with printed lyrics—activated within the asylum spaces through the pumping action of a patient or staff member's legs, and generating piano accompaniment to the lusty voices of staff and patients singing along in either segregated wards or in the recreation hall—are, in a fashion, reminiscent of karaoke. One pianola roll which formed part of a very large collection (no longer extant), used at Mayday Hills Mental Hospital, Beechworth, contains the famous 'Jealousy Tango'. The music was first used in the musical crib-sheet accompaniment of the silent film *Don Q, Son of Zoro* (1925) starring Douglas Fairbanks. It was later released as a gramophone record in the 1930s, and this instrumental piece had lyrics added to it in the late 1940s. It shot to fame with the release of Frankie Lain's version in the 1950s. A 'word roll' version of 'Jealousy Tango' (dating from after 1945 and produced by the Australian pianist Len Luscombe, who also ran the Company that released it), survives in the Museum Victoria collection.[39] The cultural specificity of this pianola roll to Australia would be replicated with other sound objects contained in psychiatric collections across the British Empire.

While the printed music that was played in the Ipswich asylum no longer survives, the music stands they would have stood on do survive. Made between the wars in the woodwork shop of the Ipswich Mental Hospital, they were used in the recreation hall and represent both a potential occupational therapy activity for a prolific woodcarving patient, and an essential component and necessary feature of musical performances. Each stand has a built-in electric light fitting and cover designed to direct the light downwards, so as to illuminate the sheet music resting below. An image of one of these stands appears in Jo Besley and Mark Finnane's chapter in this volume. Institutions mostly provided much of their own entertainment through staff efforts and the asylum band. In Australia, band members were predominantly, but not exclusively, male. In 1910 the Goodna Asylum band comprised male attendants, the medical superintendent, and one nurse, and met 'twice a week to practice between 2 and four o'clock, and they play[ed] at all the dances.' The medical superintendent observed that while there was 'one [nurse] in the band [who played cello] . . . generally the nurses do not play anything outside the piano.' For Toowoomba and Goodna asylums in Queensland musical programmes were printed in the local press. Community and professional groups also provided entertainments, and arrangements were often, but not always, made to cover their travel costs. Not all entertainment was offered with the best of intentions, however, as some visitors refused to provide the mentally ill with even an adequate standard of entertainment. In 1903 the Salvation Army Brass Band simply rehearsed rather than performed for patients. The asylum staff, clearly not impressed, took the opportunity in the annual report for that year to thank the band members for their 'disinterested efforts.'[40]

Technological advancements not only improved the quality of music provided, but also the flexibility with which it could be administered. For example, the gramophone provided a superior and consistent quality of recorded music, and readily brought the sounds of the outside world inside the institution. It also provided personal choice to staff and possibly also to patients, enabling them to tailor their listening in much the same way that we can create play lists on our computers or iPods. In the Royal Edinburgh Asylum Collection is a small early twentieth-century photograph of a male patient sitting on a veranda, intently listening to a gramophone player placed on a table. Next to the gramophone is a pile of unidentified seventy-eight revolutions per minute shellac discs. Presented here in this silent photo is an image of a patient who has the choice to listen to one of a number of other records within easy grasp. Recorded music had the added advantage of removing the reliance on staff, select patients and visitors to provide musical entertainment and hymn singing within the asylum. Whilst the titles this patient listened to at the Royal Edinburgh Asylum remain unknown, examples do survive in the southern hemisphere.

In the Australian context a selection of 78 revolutions per minute gramophone records have survived in institutional collections. The strains of music, some examples of which were over sixty years old, composed by Fritz Kreisler (1875–1962) and Antonin Dvorzák (1841–1903) were heard by patients at Beechworth, Victoria, while 'Me and my Shadow' and

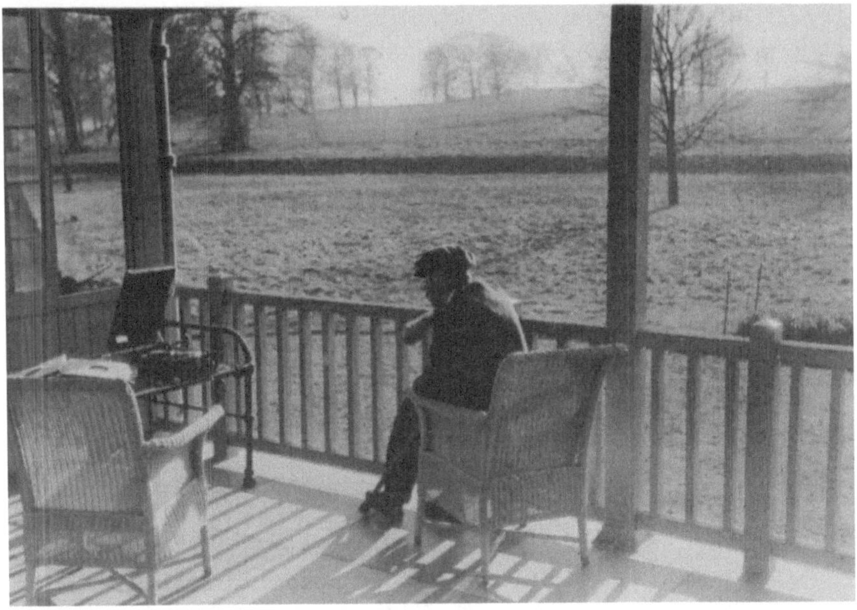

Figure 6.2 Man sitting on veranda listening to gramophone player with records on table, Royal Edinburgh Asylum, Scotland, circa 1910.
Source: Record Ref: GD16, Box 3 and reproduced by permission of the Lothian Health Services Archive, Edinburgh University Library.

'Lullaby of Broadway' from the Warner Brothers' block buster film *Gold Digger* (1935) were heard in Toowoomba, Queensland. These collections contained examples of popular and classical music sitting side-by-side. Pencil annotations such as 'good' on individual disks also indicate which items were preferred for entertainments.[41]

CONCLUSION

Psychiatric exhibits are testament to the rise and fall of the history of psychiatry, its institutions, its staff, and—to a far lesser extent—its patients. Psychiatric collections in public and restricted collections in Australia and Scotland can include a selection of recreational artefacts, ranging from gramophone records, pianola rolls, sporting trophies, and cinematographs, as well as photographs of such recreational objects. These recreation artefacts are invaluable, and each collection is specific to an individual institution and the cultural forms of gendered recreation (generic and specific) they provided. This material evidence is invaluable because it fills the large gap in the paper archives about the nature of specific forms of recreational activity—basically the many and varied ways in which recreation (religious services, hymn singing, sport, dancing and music) was used in a gendered therapeutic fashion. When played, the gramophone records recreate some of the sounds that resonated throughout the wards or recreation hall, and the sporting trophies form the tangible voice of the triumph and success of staff and patient teams in the annual community sporting competitions. This chapter has discussed why recreational items within these collections are so important, and what they represent about aspects of the soundscape of the cultural history of psychiatry in two countries from the British Empire. The gendered soundscapes from the colonial world up to the first half of the twentieth century demonstrate both continuity and change. By focusing on these recreational items in collections, the discussion offered here provides the potential for new and innovative ways of experiencing these items as sound, and moves debates well beyond just seeing objects whose primarily function and value ultimately lies in being heard.

NOTES

1. Dolly MacKinnon, "'Hearing Madness': The Soundscape of the Asylum," in *'Madness' in Australia: Histories, Heritage and the Asylum,* ed. Catharine Coleborne and Dolly MacKinnon (St. Lucia: University of Queensland Press, 2003), 73–82.
2. MacKinnon, "'Hearing Madness'," 73–82.
3. Ibid., 73–82.
4. This research forms part of my Australia Council Research Linkage Grant (2009–2012) "Reading the Objects: Developing Online Personal Stories from Australia's 'Museums of Madness', 1870–1980," with Professor Elizabeth Malcolm, University of Melbourne, and Dr Nurin Veis, Museum Victoria, and research assistants Dr Lee-Ann Monk and Dr Ann Westmore. The Museum Victoria's Psychiatric Services Collection contains over 1,646 objects from mental hospitals that operated in the state of Victoria between 1870 and 1980, and is one of the largest collections of its type in the world. This project will provide online digitized images of the objects, thus making this internationally significant collection available to a wide audience 24 hours a day.
5. MacKinnon, "'Hearing Madness'," 73–82.
6. *History and Material Culture: A Student's Guide to Approaching Sources,* ed. Karen Harvey, Routledge Guides to Using Historical Sources (London: Routledge, 2009), 1 and Preface.
7. MacKinnon, "'Hearing Madness'," 78.
8. Ibid., 78.
9. Elizabeth Willis and Karen Twigg, *Behind Closed Doors: A Catalogue of Artefacts from Victorian Psychiatric Institutions Held at Museum Victoria* (Melbourne, Victoria: Museum Victoria, 1994), 241–249, wooden sculptures and drawings, Museum Victoria, Psychiatric Services Collection, Old Registration Numbers: 721.1 [wood sculpture]; 727.1[wood sculpture]; 728.1 [wood sculpture]; 729.1[wood sculpture]; 730.1[wood sculpture]; 731.1 [wood sculpture]; 732.1 [wood sculpture]; 733.1 [wood sculpture]; 735.1 [wood sculpture]; 738.1 [drawing]; 739.1 [wood sculpture]; 741.1 [drawing]; 743.1 [wood sculpture]; 754.1 [drawing].
10. Willis and Twigg, *Behind Closed Doors,* 241.

11. *Realms of Memory: Rethinking the French Past,* ed. Pierre Nora and Lawrence D. Kritzman, trans. Arthur Goldhammer. Vol. 3: Symbols (New York: Columbia University Press, 1998), ix.
12. Dolly MacKinnon, "'Poor senseless Bess clothed in her rags and folly': Early Modern Women, Madness, and Song in Seventeenth-Century England," *Parergon* 18, no. 3 (2001): 119–151; Dolly MacKinnon, "'Hearing madness'," 73–82; Dolly MacKinnon, "'Jolly and fond of singing': The Gendered Nature of Musical Entertainment in Queensland Mental Institutions c.1870–c.1937," in *'Madness' in Australia,* ed. Coleborne and MacKinnon, 157–168; Dolly MacKinnon, "'The Trustworthy Agency of the Eyes': Reading Images of Music and Madness in Historical Context," *Health & History* 5, no. 2 (2003): 123–146; Dolly MacKinnon, "Music, Madness and the Body: Symptom and Cure," *History of Psychiatry* 17, no. 1 (2006): 9–21; Dolly MacKinnon,"'Amusements are Provided': Asylum Entertainment and Recreation in Australia and New Zealand c.1860–c.1945," in *Permeable Walls: Historical Perspectives on Hospital and Asylum Visiting,* ed. Graham Mooney and Jonathan Reinarz, Wellcome Series in the History of Medicine/ Clio Medica 86 (Amsterdam: Rodopi, 2009), 267–288.
13. *Sacred Songs & Solos: Revised and Enlarged with Standard Hymns 1200 Pieces* (London: Morgan and Scott, no date) compiled by Ira D. Sankey, cited in Dolly MacKinnon, "'A Captive Audience': Musical Concerts in Queensland Mental Institutions c.1870–c.1930", *Context* 19 (Spring 2000): 48.
14. Dolly MacKinnon, "'The Trustworthy Agency of the Eyes'," 123–146.
15. Dolly MacKinnon, "'Jolly and Fond of Singing'," in *'Madness' in Australia,* ed. Coleborne and MacKinnon, 157–168.
16. Willis and Twigg, *Behind Closed Doors*, 234, Museum Victoria, Psychiatric Services Collection, Old Registration Number: 775.1.
17. Catharine Coleborne, "Space, Power and Gender," in *'Madness' in Australia,* ed. Coleborne and MacKinnon, 56.
18. Willis and Twigg, *Behind Closed Doors,* 240, Museum Victoria, Psychiatric Services Collection, Old Registration Number: 782.1.
19. Ibid., 240, Museum Victoria, Psychiatric Services Collection, database, Registration Number: 776.1.
20. *Morningside Mirror* XX: 5 (1865), 40, Lothian Health Services Archive, Edinburgh University.
21. Lothian Health Services Archive, Edinburgh University, Box 3 GD16, Clouston Papers, [FOLDER Clouston Papers Photos REA Views], Photo B&W—Staff and patients curling; Lothian Health Services Archive, Box 3 GD16 Clouston Papers, [Folder of Photos: "Assorted Photographs"]—Photo B&W—Man sitting on veranda listening to gramophone player with records on the table.
22. *Morningside Mirror* XX: 5 (1865), 40, Lothian Health Services Archive, Edinburgh University.
23. MacKinnon, "Music, Madness and the Body," *History of Psychiatry* 17, no. 1 (2006): 9–21.
24. Mary Hutchinson and Lea Collins, "Translation: Experiments in Dialogic Representation of Cultural Diversity in Three Museum Installations," *Museum and Society* 7, no. 2 (2009): 92–109, especially 91–94.
25. Hutchinson and Collins, "Translation," 92–109, especially 91–94.
26. David Nichols, Dolly MacKinnon and Keir Reeves, "Goldfields Asylums: Anxieties, Evasions and Erasures," in *Deeper Leads: New Approaches to Victorian Goldfields History,* ed. Keir Reeves and David Nichols (Ballarat, Victoria: Ballarat Heritage Services, 2007), 39–62, and 59.
27. Hutchison and Collins "Translation," 92–109, especially 95–96.

28. MacKinnon, "'Jolly and Fond of Singing'," 167.
29. Ibid., 167.
30. Ibid., 164–166.
31. Ibid., 167.
32. Ibid., 161.
33. Willis and Twigg, *Behind Closed Doors,* 229, Museum Victoria, Psychiatric Services Collection, Old Registration Number: 717.2.
34. MacKinnon, "A Captive Audience," 43–56.
35. MacKinnon, "'Jolly and Fond of Singing'," 166.
36. Ibid., 166.
37. Ibid., 166.
38. Ibid., 166.
39. Willis and Twigg, *Behind Closed Doors,* 232, Museum Victoria, Psychiatric Services Collection, Old Registration Number: 718.3.
40. MacKinnon, "'Amusements are Provided'," 267–288.
41. MacKinnon, "'Jolly and Fond of Singing'," 166.

7 'A Grave Injustice'
The Mental Hospital and Shifting Sites of Memory

Nathan Flis and David Wright

INTRODUCTION

In 2005, a chilling story from New Westminster, British Columbia, made headlines across Canada. The British Columbia Association for Community Living, a group advocating on behalf of children and adults with intellectual disabilities, stumbled upon a large unmarked grave next to a former long-stay mental retardation facility, the Woodlands Institute.[1] After a forensic investigation, they concluded that the grounds had been the site of an institutional cemetery which had been stripped of its gravestones in order not to dismay the senior residents who had moved into one of the renovated buildings once the provincial policy of deinstitutionalisation had taken hold in the 1990s. After weeks of spadework, the volunteers began to uncover the missing gravestones. As one volunteer recalls, 'Some . . . were found in a retaining wall in a nearby ravine, some were found in walkways, and in a bizarre twist that seems to embody the indignity of the event, some were found in a barbecue pit that had been built for Woodlands staff.'[2] The experience was, for many of those involved in the restoration events, quite spiritual and symbolic: 'We weren't just touching stones, we were touching people. By recovering these headstones we're saying, "They will no longer be forgotten."'[3]

Although somewhat macabre, what eventually became the Woodlands Memorial Garden Project is hardly unique. At the Willard Asylum in New York state, for example, an internationally-acclaimed exhibition built around the abandoned suitcases of patients lamented that 'these same patients built the pine caskets, dug the graves, and made the numbered [grave] markers for these hospital cemeteries . . . '[4] Other memorials of asylum burial sites have also emerged involving the Sunbury Asylum in Victoria (Australia) and the Danvers State Hospital in Massachusetts (United States). In Australia, the Sunbury Cemetery Trust and Friends of Sunbury Cemetery worked together, in 2009, with the local newspaper under the banner, 'Marking Lost Lives', to commemorate nearly two thousand unmarked graves with the names of patients on stainless steel plaques.[5] At the Danvers State Hospital's website, under the title 'A Grave Injustice', the outrage is palpable: 'At state hospitals all across Massachusetts there is a terrible sight: row upon row of small concrete markers with only a number. These anonymous graves mark the resting place of our sisters and brothers—former patients who died at state hospitals—abandoned in life and death.'[6]

These initiatives and exhibitions, facilitated by the internet and framed by social networking sites, appear to be part of a larger trend of historicising the mental hospital. They differ in fundamental ways from previous methods of remembering the lunatic asylum, such as scholarly books on individual hospitals or the ubiquitous asylum museum run by volunteer staff and patients. The new sites of commemoration pose fascinating questions involving popular history and cultural memory that have, to date, received very little scholarly attention. This chapter, therefore, explores these new commemoration rituals and what it means for the history of mental health and psychiatry. First it will summarize trends in the historiography of memory, outlining some of the principal themes in this fascinating sub-field of modern history, in particular the memorialisation of the lives of individuals deemed to have been traumatized by war, genocide or exploitation. Second, it will examine how the recent spate of memorialisations involving mental hospitals in Canada and elsewhere have begun to eclipse asylum museums in terms of the impact on the public understanding of mental health history. Finally, the paper will analyse the implicit and explicit themes of recent commemorations which have centred on the memorialisation of asylum cemeteries, including the identification and remarking of gravesites. The chapter argues that the recent upsurge in memorialisations reflects a new era of 'remembering' and preserving the asylum (as opposed to demolishing it) and the embrace of what might be seen as a subtle new form of anti-psychiatry, where motifs borrowed from memorialisations of the Holocaust, the First World War, and American slavery are adapted to the political aspirations of 'psychiatric survivors' organisations. Aided by a sympathetic press eager to write about the 'gothic' conditions in institutions, the recent ceremonies are notable for the inclusion of senior figures of the psychiatric establishment who, for reasons of fundraising and political sensitivities, have paradoxically embraced problematic narratives of their own profession's past. The 'dark past' of institutional psychiatry is then repackaged by the psychiatric elite to show how far the psychiatric profession has progressed. These memorialisation ceremonies thus serve multiple professional, cultural and social purposes and have implications both to contemporary mental health initiatives and to our understanding of the history of mental health.

MEMORY AND MADNESS

Historians of medicine in Canada and elsewhere have largely avoided sustained engagement with what some theorists have referred to as 'cultural memory'.[7] What little has been done, has tended to be interlinked with new methodologies associated with the social history of medicine. The desire to write history 'from the patient's perspective' has given rise to a small but significant body of literature using oral interviews to reflect on the past of particular medical institutions, individual practitioners, or disease outbreaks. Perhaps more than in any other historical field, patient narratives (or patients' past experiences) have held a symbolic place in the history of madness. After all, the interrogation of memory played such a fundamental role in the development of psychological and psychiatric treatments over the course of the last century, from Freud onward.[8] Diana Gittins and Kerry Davies were among the first in the history of psychiatry to use oral interviews. In the 1990s, relying on the testimony of patients of various ages, Gittins chronicled the process of deinstitutionalisation from the Severalls Hospital in Colchester, Essex, revealing the difficulties inherent in the movement from residential to community care. Davies, on the other hand, was interested in continuities in the collective experience of residential mental patients over time; she conducted 21 interviews with former patients in Oxfordshire to assemble a larger narrative of institutional care since the introduction of the National Health Service in 1948. Two of the common 'narrative frames' that emerged from Davies' work were 'stories of loss [and] tales of survival and self-discovery.'[9]

The evolution of oral histories—of testimonies of the past—is only a small part of a larger cultural movement of remembrance. It is necessary that we examine the older attitude towards that all-important site of the history of psychiatry, the mental hospital. Pierre Nora's *Realms of Memory* was the groundbreaking work which attempted to disentangle the knotty relationship between history and memory—to do so, he focused on what he termed *lieux de mémoire*—physical spaces, or 'sites' which seemed to be the points at which the two concepts converge.[10] According to his theory, human memory recalls moments which are isolated (not necessarily bound to any context or larger picture), while history, as a precise system for describing change through time, seeks to record events in relation to each other.[11] The major difference between them is that, whereas 'history fastens upon events', memory must 'fasten upon sites'. Memory is borne of living societies, while history is detached, and always problematic in the sense that it seeks to reconstruct from dispersed fragments what no longer exists. The drawback for memory is its fleeting nature—it can only ever recall relatively recent events (within a lifetime, for example).[12] Memory, therefore, must eventually recede into history—if memories are to be preserved, they cross a threshold by being inscribed; they *become* history.

In the historiography of madness, the mental institution has, for more than half a century, been the central *lieu de mémoire* around which most of the history of psychiatry has been constructed. Michel Foucault's *Madness and Civilization,* the landmark treatise against which most historical accounts are somehow compared, was undoubtedly influenced by the French trajectory of thought that emerged from Maurice Halbswach's idea of 'collective memory' and Jacques Lacan's theory of the 'social imaginary'.[13] Foucault began his book by invoking the image of the medieval Ship of Fools, a distant memory that haunted the collective European psyche, of 'mad men' being loaded onto merchant ships to be transported to distant lands so that the cities would be rid of them—a sort of mobile proto-asylum. For Foucault, the ship represented the inability of western society to cope in a humane way with its mentally ill (and the horrific nature of madness itself), a tradition that from the seventeenth century onwards, gave way to the coercive incarceration and treatment of mad individuals, ultimately culminating in the nineteenth-century public lunatic asylum.[14]

For most historians and non-historians, the asylum also constitutes the centrepiece of popular memory about society's engagement (or rejection) of the mad. In the second half of the twentieth century, many of the mental hospitals originally constructed in Victorian Canada and elsewhere were often rebuilt because, as one senior psychiatrist put it, they were 'highly visible reminder(s) of a previous era of treatment of the mentally ill from which, thankfully, we have emerged'.[15] The original edifice of the Toronto Asylum, which will be discussed at greater length, was largely demolished in the winter of 1975. A former patient of the institution (later the Queen Street Mental Hospital, which was located at 999 Queen Street West) saw demolition as the only solution to the building which embodied a remembered past that was painful. Joan Sutton, a writer, was rather poetic:

> 999: I will never forget those haunted faces, haunted eyes, neglected bodies, and forgotten spirits.
>
> 999: rows of old people, plopped there because there was no where else to go, no one who wanted them, the debris of a society that values only youth, a world that neglects to nourish its roots . . .
>
> There were the sights: barbaric reminders of human indignity, human indifference, callousness.
>
> But mostly, 999 was a smell . . . If you were there once, you would not need to preserve the building: You would never forget it. I can sit here now, surrounded by light and warmth and companionship and recreate that monstrous building, even though it is years since I was there.[16]

In most accounts written in the 1970s, the image of the nineteenth-century asylum was blurred with the mental hospital of the early to mid-twentieth century—that is, institutions like the one described in Ken Kesey's novel *One Flew Over the Cuckoo's Nest* (1962), a highly influential account of life in an American mental hospital in part based on Kesey's own experience of working as an attendant in a California state institution in the 1950s. It is no coincidence that during this time, philosophers and sociologists (such as Michel Foucault and Erving Goffman), and some ex-members of the psychiatric profession (such as R. D. Laing and Thomas Szasz) penned the first critiques and stories of institutionalisation from different perspectives—a body of work that came to be known as the first wave of the anti-psychiatry movement. Their collective ideas focused on several aspects of modern psychiatry—the institutions themselves, the nature of involuntary confinement, and the experimental treatments of the mid-twentieth century. Their influence can be seen in scholarly works highly critical of the rise of the asylum, such as David J. Rothman's *The Discovery of the Asylum* and Andrew Scull's *Museums of Madness*.[17] The unrelenting critique of mental institutions in the 1960s and 1970s was accompanied by the establishment of small sites of remembrance; the mental hospital museum.

MUSEUMS OF MADNESS

It is noteworthy that all four of the provincial mental hospitals in the province of Ontario that date back to the nineteenth century had, at one time, an archive or museum, or at least rooms that were seconded to perform the function of a museum. In the Toronto Asylum (by then the Queen Street Mental Health Centre), the Archives for the History of Canadian Psychiatry and Mental Health Services was created in 1982; originally, it consisted of rooms full of old ECT machines, uncatalogued manuscripts, and other miscellany. The volunteer organization called itself the Friends of the Museum of Mental Health, even though, in fact, no Museum *per se* existed. As the institution was annexed by a larger mental health non-profit corporation, known as the Centre for Addiction and Mental Health (CAMH), the group was restyled as the Friends of the CAMH Archives. Regular rotating displays now combine reproductions of photographs of the former institution and staff members with artefacts such as staff uniforms. Assembled by volunteers, these displays are mounted in lit glass cases in the lobby and hallway near the entrance to the CAMH Queen Street site; they share space with—and perhaps gain some relevance from—being juxtaposed with art by former and current patients.

In the Kingston Psychiatric Hospital (the former Kingston Asylum), four exhibits contain a variety of artefacts related to the history of the asylum.[18] The first, A Time of Transition: Mental Illness and Rockwood Asylum in the 1800s, contains a lock and key, and a hammer used in the original asylum, as well as postcards c.1905. The second case, Patients and Life at the Museum, displays a bowling trophy from 1923, a saddle stitching clamp c.1900, a woodworking plane and blade, and a doily possibly made by a patient in the early 1900s. In the third exhibit, The Staff at Rockwood, are a reproduction of a nurse's uniform from the 1890s and a reproduction of a nursing student's notebook from 1907. The final exhibit, Changing Treatments for Mental Illness, contains a scarificator from the 1800s, a syringe from the 1890s, a trepanning set c.1890, a bath thermometer from the 1900s, and a pharmacy case from the late 1800s. This motley assortment of items evokes a kind of morbid fascination for some; others may see these objects as reminders of a dark past. The narrative structure of the museum, however, and the historical message, appear to be fragmented and ambiguous.

In London, what was known as an Archival and Teaching Museum was established in 1970 at the London Psychiatric Hospital (formerly the London Asylum), what would later be known as St. Joseph's Regional Mental Health Care London (RMHCL). The collection had been used as an educational resource for psychiatry and psychology postgraduate programs at the University of Western Ontario (also in London) and allied health care professionals, and was also open for public viewing. In this way the Museum had the didactic purpose of representing a history of psychiatric services for a generation of future professionals and the public alike. In December 2008, the photographic and archival collection was donated to the Archival and Research Collections Center at the University of Western Ontario, and the artefacts to Museum London, the general city museum. An exhibit called Cultivating Care, based on the acquired items, was on display at Museum London from January to May 2009.

A museum has existed at the site of the former Hamilton Asylum since about the time that, like Toronto, the Hamilton Asylum was demolished and new modern facilities were erected on the same physical site. A recent brochure rather dryly describes a 'collection of documents, photographs and artifacts pertaining to the history of psychiatric treatment in the Province of Ontario, from 1876 (the first year of the institution) to 1976. Activities include tours of the museum, presentations to medical disciplines on early psychiatric care and treatment, an annual Christmas open house and participation in community-wide events at the hospital.'[19] The current brochure, however, certainly does no justice to the bizarre selection of items to be found there, including a mannequin wearing a nurse's outfit, an old wheelchair, games used by former patients (worn playing cards and an old cribbage board), a government-approved oak easy chair (heavy enough so that it could not be picked up and thrown), leather wrist restraints, a tub used for hydrotherapy (or dunking), an irrigation syringe, surgical tools such as a circular trephine (for boring holes in the skull to relieve hydrocephalic pressure), a preserved slice of the brain of a child with hydroencephaly, a 'Utica crib'—an oblong wooden crate with a lid (apparently used to hold hysterical patients, named for the Utica Asylum in New York State, where the box design originated), and a mid-twentieth century machine called the 'Reiter Sedac Stimulator' used to administer ECT. Nevertheless, the Museum, established and run by a small group of volunteers (many of whom are staff or former staff) purports to preserve the history of psychiatric treatment for professionals and the public.[20]

At a time when McMaster University and St Joseph's Healthcare Hamilton (currently the non-profit corporation with responsibility for the successor to the Hamilton Psychiatric Hospital) has secured provincial funds for a new psychiatric facility, the representations of the history of the site have become increasingly important. Recently commenting on the in-house museum, Dr Robert Zipursky, the Chair of Psychiatry at McMaster University (also in Hamilton) and Chief of Psychiatry at St Joseph's Healthcare, affirms that it is

> '. . . very important, as we look at developing views of mental illness in the future, to be in touch with the past and the progress we've made in the past 130 years . . . There have been dramatic changes in the field and I hope we'll see a whole new way of understanding mental illness.'[21]

It is worth mentioning something here about the phenomenon of these museums of madness. There is certainly nothing personal about the types of artefacts displayed. Rather, they seem to be voyeuristic in their insistence that the history of madness is one of violence and trauma; they implicitly neglect and victimise (and even make invisible) the patient rather than empower him or her, which is precisely antithetical to the aims of the new forms of commemoration. Few appear to have been as nuanced and balanced as the Museum of Brisbane's Remembering Goodna exhibition in Australia in 2009.[22] Doubtless, some of the objects in these institutional collections have fascinating provenances and stories to tell. As Catharine Coleborne has done for the Australian context, it is worth asking the questions of what intentions such collections serve, and what can be done to revitalise them so that they speak meaningfully to the history of madness.[23]

From the 1970s until the end of the twentieth century the asylum museum was the dominant site for remembering the lunatic asylum and, by implication, the history of mental health and psychiatry. These initiatives arose, in part, as a collective institutional reaction to the downsizing of long-stay mental hospitals and the desire for volunteers to erect modest museums to preserve hospital memories. The results were, however, strangely depersonalised, bereft of the experiences and meanings of patients themselves. In recent years, however, there has been a demonstrable shift in the site and nature of remembering the mental hospital, from the ubiquitous asylum museums to more diverse and public acts of remembrance organised by patients' groups. It is not a coincidence that these new commemoration ceremonies have reached a crescendo at another moment in history when the physical structures of the old mental hospitals are being destroyed, refashioned or repurposed. These ceremonies represent shifting sites of remembrance that have implications for our memory of the asylum and the public's understanding of the history of mental health and psychiatry.

ANOTHER BRICK IN THE WALL

The former Toronto Asylum serves as an excellent case study of these shifting sites of remembrance. In Canada's largest city there have been a series of events to commemorate what remains of the perimeter wall of the institution, originally built as the provincial asylum in the late 1840s. As mentioned above, the Toronto Asylum for the Insane was dismantled in the mid-1970s to make way for a 'modern' psychiatric facility, which was ultimately renamed the Queen Street Mental Health Centre. Despite considerable opposition from some architectural historians, the old asylum buildings in Toronto were destroyed, partly in response to the dilapidated state of the old structures, but also as a self-conscious political statement against the older generation of long-stay mental hospitals. Unlike Britain, where the National Trust system ensured the preservation of most of the Victorian asylum structures as Grade 1 or 2 listed buildings, the much less comprehensive system of designating heritage buildings in Canada (whereby each building must be assessed upon petition and designated a heritage building by a municipal government) did not ensure the survival of the original asylum buildings. Of course, there is not always agreement about what exactly should be preserved; Victorian asylums in the British world were grand, complex properties with many outbuildings, gardens, and even farms and shops. In the Australian context, Dolly MacKinnon demonstrates how the battles to preserve individual institutions are more often than not quite idiosyncratic. Using the reconfiguration and renovation of the Kew Cottages in Victoria and the Challinor Centre in Queensland as examples, MacKinnon exposes the difficulty with heritage laws, that sometimes only buildings of a particular age are preserved to the detriment and destruction of others—we are then left with what she calls 'partial histories.'[24]

In Toronto, the 'modern' facilities of the 1970s are now themselves being razed to the ground as part of a multi-year, radical re-visioning of the psychiatric landscape in the west-central part of the city. To coincide with this multi-million dollar reconstruction project, the new managers of the site—the University of Toronto-affiliated Centre for Addition and Mental Health (CAMH)—have hosted well-publicised fundraising and 'awareness-raising' events, jointly organised with patients' advocacy groups. Some of these events have focused on memorialisation events related to the remaining asylum wall. Public auctions of some of the bricks (for fundraising purposes) as well as commemorative plaques on the remaining sections have been widely publicised in local newspapers.[25] For many of the former patients, the wall is charged with meaning. According to the Director of the Psychiatric Survivors Association of Toronto (PSAT), Geoffrey Reaume, who has also published a book on the history of the patients in what was once Canada's largest psychiatric institution, the inmates built it with 'unpaid' labour in the nineteenth century.[26] The allusion to slave labour—as in the war-time camps during World War II or in Communist

China labour colonies—drives home the point of exploitation as a central theme in the history of the mental hospital. The cultural references to other late twentieth-century momentous historical events—such as the destruction of the Berlin Wall (pieces of which were taken as totems by protesters, others purchased as commemorative pieces)—could hardly escape people's attention. In a sense, the bricks have become pneumonic devices for the history of the mental hospital itself.

The unusual alliance between PSAT and the psychiatric elite of CAMH reflects several fascinating convergences. First, PSAT, once a loosely organized group of former patients often voicing the more extreme versions of anti-psychiatry, has matured over the last two decades to become a well-organised advocacy organisation. The group has supplemented patient-led theatre and social events with public tours of the grounds of the former Toronto asylum led often by Reaume himself. On his tour of the grounds, Reaume points out the remaining portions of the wall; he talks about the patients tilling the earth in their allotments; he refers to other surviving architectural elements such as the wooden spiral staircase that originally led up to the front/central water tower; and he takes tours to a limestone brick outbuilding of c.1860 which housed laundry facilities used by some of the earliest patients. All of these sites of memory invoke the labour and isolation of patients, perhaps none more than the dedication of the remaining portion of the patient-built asylum wall. The allusions to unpaid labour also invoke suggestions of plantation work by slaves prior to emancipation. Abolitionist references are not far from the surface. At the Willard Asylum across the border in New York state, the commemoration of which has been assisted by PSAT member Gayle Hornstein, who compiled a bibliography of over 600 first-person patient narratives, believes that 'patient memoirs are a kind of protest literature, like slave narratives or witness testimonies.'[27]

Another group of activists connected to the memory of the former Toronto Asylum is called the 'Angels of 999', led by an activist named Ruth Stackhouse, and mainly composed of those who were once or are still treated at CAMH. This group is credited with writing a song and staging a play dedicated to the wall, and by association, paying tribute to those who built it. All of this creative activity surrounded the movement to preserve the few remaining parts of the asylum which were at risk in the latest plans to renovate. In the spring of 2010, there was a silent auction that included bricks from the crumbling or unsalvageable portions of the 'patient-built' wall. The bricks sold were no longer bare; they had been painted by various members of the community—here we have a memorialising process at work: a unique interaction between the living who are interested in knowing and remembering with those objects which in themselves have come to symbolise the wall as a whole (and by association, the entire asylum), as well as patient labour and struggle. These endeavors continue, so there is an unfolding history of remembering to be written. The wall is therefore a site of remembrance, for speaking to lost generations, an inspiration for art, and a meeting place for activists.

Those familiar with the long and tense relationship between psychiatric 'survivors' (or 'consumers') and the psychiatric profession might notice an unusual alliance over recent acts of commemoration. As the cultural theorist Marita Sturken reminds us, 'What memories tell us, more than anything, is of the stakes held by individuals and institutions in attributing meaning to the past.'[28] In part this is due to the fact that the stakes for the psychiatric leadership in Toronto are huge. The $400 million (Canadian) renovation of the Queen Street West site in Toronto has launched an unprecedented alliance between the psychiatric administrators and the very organisation that had been denouncing much of psychiatric practice as 'inhumane' and 'exploitative' for the past four decades. Paul Garfinkel, a psychiatrist and CEO of CAMH, states rather ambiguously that the multi-year plan to thoroughly remake the Queen Street site '[is] a bold thing to do and the right thing to do. We have mistreated these people, and they deserve a humane and caring society and treatment.'[29] Although it is not clear whether the 'we' stands for society in general or the mental health professions in particular, the nod to the 'mistreatment' of the mentally ill in the past is clear. His positioning is, by necessity, a delicate balancing act. The asylum grounds—no longer on the edge of Victorian Toronto but rather now in the increasingly trendy central west of the city—will see even the 1970s structures demolished and replaced with contemporary multi-purpose buildings. Once a downtrodden area of halfway houses and low-end coffee shops, the Queen Street and Ossington Street area around the former asylum is now becoming a highly fashionable and up-and-coming part of town. Streets that formerly ended at the gates of the asylum grounds will cut through the former site, creating a new twenty-seven-acre 'urban oasis' or 'urban village' of mental health services, mixed with restaurants, condominiums and boutiques. Thus, paradoxically, the rise in the commemorative plaques and tours in Toronto may well be accompanied by the slow decline of what Michael J. Dear and Jennifer R. Wolch once famously described as the 'psychiatric ghetto'–the physical space of inner-city residences near psychiatric facilities that housed former patients and other marginalised individuals.[30] Thus the rise of commemoration may, somewhat ironically, be accompanied by the decline in the sense of ownership of the area by the mentally ill themselves. As Reaume wryly observes: 'We have to make sure that they [former patients] are part of the [new] community and not shunned.'[31]

Although there has been much publicity around the asylum wall commemorations, PSAT has also been active in reclaiming cemeteries, as witnessed by their most recent initiative, the Lakeshore Asylum Cemetery Project. The mandate is to recover and create memorials for the over 1,500 unmarked graves in Etobicoke (just east of Toronto), which belong to patients of the former Mimico Insane Asylum, a former branch institution of the Toronto asylum.[32] The focus on gravesites borrows from several dominant cultural motifs in the second half of the twentieth century. The rhetoric of commemoration involving involuntary residents invokes tropes of Holocaust remembrance and (most relevant to recent Canadian public memory), the scandal of the Indian Residential Schools.[33] Such allusions to the Holocaust are reinforced with an older anti-psychiatry critique that equates the involuntary treatment of patients as tantamount to medical experimentation and torture. In this way, the crude anti-psychiatry critiques of the 1970s have given way to more subtle and pervasive cultural references to major traumatic events in history. Their memory borrows from cultural tropes of trauma and victimisation as evidenced in allusions to the Holocaust. The focus on cemeteries also invokes associations with the dead of the two world wars, a reverential trope in many western countries that is beyond critique. The cemetery projects thus serve important social and political, as well as cultural ends. On one level they provide a necessary and dignified service—culturally validated by the public at large—to clean up and properly designate graves. They also provide a forum for collective action which provides meaning and helps define new patient advocacy groups. On a more abstract level, the new cemeteries afford an opportunity where survivors can 'speak' to the dead.

CONCLUSIONS

In the 1970s, many of the provincial asylums in Canada and elsewhere underwent a radical transformation. As deinstitutionalisation took hold and the critique of long-stay mental hospitals was reaching a crescendo, provincial authorities began to radically reorganise the old residential asylum buildings. Many were torn down and replaced with new 'modern' facilities oriented to outpatient care. As other chapters in this volume have suggested, the closure or downsizing of mental hospitals precipitated in-house voluntary initiatives such as the formation of in-house museums as a way of preserving the history of these remarkable institutions. The museums were, for a generation, one of the principal ways of remembering the asylum, providing a site in which the general public could form views about the history of the mental hospital. In many ways, a new wave of re-visioning the mental hospital is taking hold across North America, resulting in the buildings constructed in the 1970s now being destroyed and replaced by newer institutions. One might suppose that the newer initiatives of commemoration, discussed previously, have also been precipitated by the new wave of mental hospital reconfiguration, as hospital administrators—eager to distance themselves from the public memory of the Victorian asylum—seek to engage in a difficult historical discussion of the social function of these controversial institutions.

The new commemoration events, and the no doubt sincere desire of administrators to construct new buildings that would not perpetuate the stigma associated with mental illness, may well reconfigure the relationship between society and the mentally ill. One could argue, in fact, that the relationship between the mental hospital and the public has come full circle. Janet Miron and others have demonstrated how, in the first generation of operation, the Victorian mental hospital was a site of public knowledge and education (as well as spectacle), as tourists regularly visited these large public institutions to witness the state of mental illness and its treatment.[34] Amongst the many justifications for keeping the asylums open to the public was the strong didactic purpose.[35] However, by the early twentieth century, medical superintendents by and large managed to slowly close off the asylum to visitors, citing privacy and distraction as the principal reasons to prevent the inflow of outsiders. This led to the greater isolation of the public mental hospitals from society at large. Paradoxically, the commemoration events can be seen, on one level, as a re-engagement of the general public with mental health issues and treatment. On the other hand, they tend to confuse periodisation in history; the public all too often misattributes the medical experimentation of the early to mid-twentieth century with the first two generations of the asylum in the nineteenth.[36]

The communities of volunteers that have emerged are also forging an identity for themselves, as much as they are restoring identities to the too-often faceless former patients whose lives they are memorialising. These new initiatives have received little or no scholarly attention; indeed, some of them are described for the first time in this paper. One of the reasons for this is the time it has taken for psychiatric 'consumer' and 'survivor' movements to coalesce, establish a membership, and forge an agenda. As Barbara Everett points out (and Everett appears to be unique in investigating the nature of their efforts), such groups take years, even decades to gather momentum, to build a strong agenda, and raise a collective voice.[37] Eventually, perhaps, the formation and growing pains of such groups will have its own history. The new voice—one of remembering, preserving, and the forging of identity—is one of the most interesting developments to emerge in the debate over what constitutes the history of madness.

The implications for the public understanding of mental health and psychiatry, however, are complicated. The participation of leading psychiatrists and administrators in these events—which, as suggested before, are replete with images that are profoundly problematic and critical of psychiatry's past–threaten to reinforce popular prejudices about psychiatric practice and stereotypes about involuntary treatment. Deeply sensitive to accusations of past malpractice and abuses, psychiatrists are now engaged in an awkward cohabitation with groups that frequently equate their forefathers as heartless scientific experimenters. Moreover, for historians of psychiatry, the focus on cemeteries and the remaining edifices of the old mental hospitals occludes the scholarship over the last generation which has revealed the permeability of the mental hospital, one factor of which was the discharge of many patients back into the community where they largely vanished from the public record. The stereotype then of 'out of mind, out of sight' is simply reinforced in the cultural memory. The plurality of experiences and the continued engagement of many families receive little or no attention in these new commemorations. They raise public awareness and interest in the history of madness, but do so using tropes that do no justice to the incredible complexity of the relationship between society and the mad over the course of the last 200 years.

NOTES

1. The Woodlands institute began life as the Provincial Asylum for the Insane, New Westminster, British Columbia (1878). Over time, a newer facility was built in Coquitlam (Riverdale Hospital) and the New Westminster institution began to focus increasingly on the 'mentally retarded'. It was officially repurposed in 1950 as the Woodlands School/Institute, a residential facility for the developmentally disabled. See http://www.bcmhas.ca/AboutUs /History.htm.
2. As quoted in Mark Hume, "Giving dignity to the dead B.C. tried to hide from view," *The Globe and Mail*, July 18, 2005, page A01.
3. Ibid.
4. http://suitcaseexhibit.org/indexhasflash.html (accessed August 1, 2010).
5. "Sunbury asylum memorial plans on track, Hume Council says", *Sunbury Leader* (Australia); online version http://sunbury-leader.whereilive.com.au/news/story/sunbury-asylum-memorial-plans-on-track-city/, dated 22 January 09 (accessed August 1, 2010).
6. The Danvers (Massachusetts) State Memorial Committee webpage: http://dsmc.info/ (accessed August 6, 2010).
7. For an application of the theory of cultural memory to recent commemorations of traumatic events in American history, see Marita Sturken, *Tangled Memories: The Vietnam War, the AIDS Epidemic, and the Politics of Remembering* (Berkeley: University of California Press, 1997).
8. For a greater examination of memory and trauma within historical scholarship, see *Traumatic Pasts: History, Psychiatry, and Trauma in Modern Age, 1870–1930,* ed. Mark S. Micale and Paul Lerner (Cambridge: Cambridge University Press, 2001) and *Trauma and Memory: Reading, Healing, and Making Law,* ed. Austin Sarat, Nadav Davidovitch, and Michal Alberstein (Stanford: Stanford University Press, 2007).
9. Kerry Davies, '"Silent and Censured Travellers'? Patients' Narratives and Patients' Voices: Perspectives on the History of Mental Illness since 1948," *Social History of Medicine* 14, no. 2 (2001): 267–292; Diana Gittins, *Madness in Its Place: Narratives of Severalls Hospital, 1913–1997* (London: Routledge, 1998).
10. Pierre Nora, "Between Memory and History: *Les Lieux de Mémoire*," *Representations* 26 (1989): 7–25.
11. Jacques Le Goff and Pierre Nora, eds., *Constructing the Past: Essays in Historical Methodology* (Cambridge: Cambridge University Press, 1985); Pierre Nora and Lawrence D. Kritzman, *Realms of Memory,* 3 vols., trans. Arthur Goldhammer (New York: Columbia University Press, 1996–1998); Pierre

Nora, ed., *Rethinking France: Les Lieux de Mémoire,* 2 vols., trans. Mary Seidman Trouille and David P. Jordan (Chicago: Chicago University Press, 2001).

12. Nora was reacting against the predominant academic view that memory (as a popular notion of past events) was inferior to historical scholarship; he relied heavily on Halbswachs, but he was also part of a new generation of revisionist historians of which his colleague Jacques Le Goff was an important contributor. For Le Goff's classic treatise on memory and history, see *Histoire et Mémoire* (Paris: Gallimard, 1988).
13. Maurice Halbwachs, *On Collective Memory*, trans. Lewis A. Coser (Chicago: University of Chicago Press, 1992); Jacques Lacan, *The Four Fundamental Concepts of Psychoanalysis,* ed. Jacques-Alain Miller, trans. Alan Sheridan (New York: Norton, 1988). In his investigation of the origins of modernity, the Canadian philosopher Charles Taylor extended Lacan's definition of the social imaginary from a cluster of ideas and beliefs to that which 'enables . . . the practices of society' to make sense of this group of ideas and beliefs. Charles Taylor, *Modern Social Imaginaries* (Durham: Duke University Press, 2004).
14. Michel Foucault, *Madness and Civilisation: A History of Madness in the Age of Reason,* trans. Richard Howard (New York: Routledge, 2001).
15. These are the words of Frederick Lowy, chairman of the University of Toronto's Department of Psychiatry in the mid 1970s. See George Baird, researched by Robert Hill, "999 Queen: A Case Study of Government Demolition," in *The Second City Book: Studies of Urban and Suburban Canada,* ed. James Lorimer and Evelyn Ross (Toronto: James Lorimer and Company, 1977), 75.
16. Joan Sutton, "Sutton's Place: Column by Joan Sutton," *Toronto Sun*, December 17, 1975. Reproduced in Lorimer and Ross, *The Second City Book*, 74.
17. Andrew Scull, *Museums of Madness: The Social Organisation of Insanity in Nineteenth-Century England* (London: Allen Lane, 1979); David J. Rothman, *The Discovery of the Asylum: Social Order and Disorder in the New Republic* (Boston: Little Brown, 1971).
18. The Kingston Asylum was also known, from time to time, as Rockwood, or the Rockwood Asylum.
19. Brochure, Hamilton Psychiatric Hospital Museum, c.1990.
20. Hamilton Psychiatric Hospital Museum, at http://www.inform.hamilton.ca/record/HAM0610? UseCICVw=43; or http://www.stjosham.on.ca.
21. Bob Zipursky, "Museum has shocking artifacts: Psychiatric hospital collection includes brain stimulator and wrist restraints," *The Hamilton Spectator*, August 28, 2010.
22. Fiona Paisley, "Peeling Back History: The Remembering Goodna Exhibition", Exhibition Review, *Health & History* 11, no. 1 (2009).
23. Catharine Coleborne, "Collecting 'Madness': Psychiatric Collections and the Museum in Victoria and Western Australia,' in *'Madness' in Australia: Histories, Heritage and the Asylum,* ed. Catharine Coleborne and Dolly MacKinnon (St. Lucia: Queensland University Press, 2003), 184.
24. Dolly MacKinnon, "The 20th-century Mental Hospital: A place in history but not in the adaptive reuse of surviving built heritage environments," paper presented at *Green Fields, Brown Fields, New Fields*, the 10th Australasian Urban History, Planning History Conference, University of Melbourne, 7–10 February 2010, 359–367.
25. See for example Leslie Scrivener, "Breakout at the Asylum: How a radical $400 million rebuilding of the Centre for Addiction and Mental Health will make it a central part of the Queen West Community," *Toronto Star*, February 25, 2007, Front Cover and A8.

26. Geoffrey Reaume, *Remembrance of Patients Past: Patient Life at the Toronto Hospital for the Insane, 1870–1940* (Don Mills: Oxford University Press, 2000); also Reaume, "Patients at Work: Insane Asylum Inmates' Labour in Ontario, 1841–1900," in *Mental Health and Canadian Society: Historical Perspectives*, ed. James E. Moran and David Wright (Montreal and Kingston: McGill-Queen's University Press, 2006), 69–96.
27. See the online version of the exhibit, at http://suitcaseexhibit.org/ (accessed August 1, 2010).
28. Sturken, *Tangled Memories*, 9.
29. Leslie Scrivener, "Breaking down barriers on Queen Street W: After 157 years, the most daring redevelopment in CAMH's history has begun," *Toronto Star*, February 25, 2007, A8–9.
30. Michael J. Dear and Jennifer R. Wolch, *Landscapes of Despair: From Deinstitutionalization to Homelessness* (Princeton: Princeton University Press, 1987).
31. Ibid.
32. Details about the Lakeshore Asylum Cemetery Project can be found at http://www. psychiatricsurvivor archives.com/cemetery/index.html.
33. Throughout most of the first half of the twentieth century, the Canadian government coordinated a program—often run by local religious denominations—to forcibly take Native Canadian and Inuit children from their families and force them to go hundreds of miles from their homes to be educated in residential schools. This was part of the process of racial assimilation and the civilizing process of the European Canadians. This phenomenon, with parallels in Australia and New Zealand, was riddled with physical and sexual abuse that took decades to be taken seriously by the Canadian government and general public. The memory of the residential schools has now taken the form of a Truth and Reconciliation commission modeled on the South African tribunal of the same name.
34. Janet Miron, "'Open to the Public': Touring Ontario Asylums in the Nineteenth Century," in Moran and Wright, 19–48. Miron, Coleborne, and MacKinnon all address this issue in their respective chapters in *Permeable Walls: Historical Perspectives on Hospital and Asylum Visiting*, ed. Graham Mooney and Jonathan Reinarz (Amsterdam: Rodopi, 2009).
35. Janet Miron, "'In View of the Knowledge to be Acquired': Public Visits to New York's Asylums in the Nineteenth Century," in Mooney and Reinarz, 243–266.
36. We are grateful to the editors for this insightful observation.
37. Barbara Everett, "Something is Happening: The Contemporary Consumer and Psychiatric Survivor Movement in Historical Context," *Journal of Mind and Behavior* 15, nos. 1 and 2 (1994): 55–70.

8 Remembering Goodna

Stories from a Queensland Mental Hospital

Joanna Besley and Mark Finnane

A museum exhibition is most often thought of as a conclusion—an encapsulation of a subject, neatly and attractively presented and brought to a close, designed so that visitors can comfortably access and absorb a topic. In this chapter, we instead consider the generative potential of exhibitions. We examine the idea that an exhibition can be an active gathering, a process that creates collections rather than just draws from them. If curators and others work closely and collaboratively with individuals and communities who have a personal stake in the history being presented in exhibitions, then memories, stories, fragments and even absences—not just objects—become essential elements of both collections and exhibitions. The potential returns of this approach are significant, although it also challenges the way that museums and curators have traditionally worked. This is particularly true of exhibitions and collections that represent the troubling history of psychiatry and the experience of being institutionalised, something that those who have never experienced mental illness themselves can only ever partially comprehend. Exhibiting personally remembered versions of the past and working together with people who have experienced multiple traumas and distress is complex, and comes with heightened responsibilities. As Gaynor Kavanagh asserts, 'when museums actively engage with the personal, what is discovered is that the work is neither straightforward nor anticipated—just like memory itself. Working with memories implicitly means working with emotions . . . It is not easy . . . Such work tests the limitations as well as the potential of museum professionals and museum practice . . . This is never more true than when memories of trauma are stimulated. When this occurs nothing less than a serious reassessment, and, if need be, realignment of museum work is required.'[1]

This chapter will unpack the 'realignment' Kavanagh describes by critically reflecting upon the exhibition Remembering Goodna: Stories From a Queensland Mental Hospital, presented by Museum of Brisbane (MoB) from November 2007 to March 2008.[2] The curatorial approach to the exhibition will be appraised, alongside a significant new documentary collection that was created throughout the exhibition from over 600 written comments made by visitors.[3] We also examine how memories and stories from community participants deepened the interpretation and visitor experience of the collections featured in the exhibition, as well as considerably expanding the collections themselves.

In keeping with the disability movement's ethos of 'Nothing About Us Without Us',[4] Remembering Goodna was developed collaboratively with past and present staff and patients of the hospital as well as their family, friends and allies. This collaboration and the practice of community collections—of locating and interpreting personal and non-institutional collections—drove the curatorial approach. The exhibition also built upon historical research conducted during a project between Griffith University and Queensland Health, with funding support from the Australian Research Council involving extensive archival research and oral history. Thus, grounded in a foundation of historical evidence and supplemented by powerful processes of collective and individual remembering, the exhibition was able to bring to life the history of this significant institution and engage the community in a dialogue about difference, wellness and belonging, both now and in the past.

HISTORY AT THE MARGINS

> Having been to The Park and seen the old buildings there I was haunted by what must have gone on. This is a very important exhibition because it acknowledges the pain and suffering those people went through. It must not be kept behind closed doors. Finally it has come out into the open. It is important not to forget what went on there. I was inspired by the bravery of former patients who talked of their experiences. My heart goes out to them and all the people still living either at The Park or in isolation in the community.
>
> Female visitor aged 25[5]

Remembering Goodna explored the intricate and difficult history of Queensland's oldest and largest mental hospital, situated on an isolated site at Goodna on the Brisbane River, halfway between the cities of Brisbane and Ipswich. Its location and history articulates the long-standing impetus to relegate mental illness to the margins. Founded in 1865 as Woogaroo Lunatic Asylum, the institution has been known by a succession of names. In the late nineteenth century it became Goodna Hospital for the Insane, then Mental Hospital Goodna, then Brisbane Special Hospital, then Wolston Park Hospital, and now, The Park Centre for Mental Health, each name reflecting a constant aspiration to escape the stigma associated with an institution for 'the insane'.[6] In the exhibition, the place was referred to simply as 'Goodna', which is how it was known in Queensland for many years—local idiom for asylum, with 'going up the line to Goodna' a threat that needed no translation. From an isolated colonial asylum, one of the very first public institutions maintained by the newly self-governing colony of Queensland, through the creation of an idealised environment based on notions of moral therapy, the consolidation of medical knowledge through the mental hygiene movement and then a long period of deinstitutionalisation from the post-war period to today, its history charts changing ideas about the treatment of mental illness over the past two centuries.[7]

Patients came to Goodna from all over Queensland and their numbers increased rapidly during the life of the institution, with more than 50,000 people admitted over its duration. Such a substantial institution had a correspondingly large staff. The place was a self-contained community with a close symbiotic relationship to the adjoining township (later, suburb) of Goodna where most of the staff lived. For many locals, the hospital was the place of employment for generations of the same family. The site was farmed and even sustained some profitable production, while a large team of carpenters, plumbers, blacksmiths, engineers and other tradesmen kept the place running, including the generation of electricity from a sizeable powerhouse. Strikingly, the institution was also the product of the labor of its inmates, as patients worked in all areas of the hospital's operations until the 1940s, their labour coming to an end in the post-war years as a result of the agitation of trade unions, the development of psychotherapeutic drugs, and the gradual onset of deinstitutionalisation.[8]

From 1909, an English-trained psychiatrist, H. Byam Ellerton, transformed the Goodna site into its modern form. There was a utopian element to Ellerton's vision, one that sought to capture the potential of an integrated, almost self-sufficient community. The grounds became gardens and meal times became opportunities for the social improvement and rehabilitation of patients in dining rooms resembling Edwardian tea-rooms, with small tables in place of benches and mess tables, pictures on the wall and potted palms on sideboards. Yet for all this, the institution was over-crowded, short of qualified staff and lacking in adequate Government funding or interest. A patient who was not released within a year of admission had a high likelihood of staying many years, perhaps the rest of their life, short or long as that might be. The institutionalisation of those with mental illness in Queensland became an efficient system of control and regulation with an emphasis on confinement rather than treatment or care. By the mid-1950s Goodna was the largest single mental hospital in Australia, with about 2,500 daily average residents and a staff of nearly 800.[9]

With the worldwide move to de-institutionalisation, the hospital's population fell rapidly from the 1970s although as late as 1990 the institution remained one of the largest psychiatric facilities in Australia. Over ten years, reforms determined by the National Mental Health Policy were implemented and Wolston Park Hospital formally closed in 2001, to be succeeded on site by The Park Centre for Mental Health. No more than 190 people are now accommodated at The Park. Buildings have been demolished and new buildings reflect contemporary treatment strategies. Patients, now known as consumers, live in small group homes or individual units and many do their own cooking, cleaning and washing. As one former patient described it in the exhibition, the place 'is a ghost of its former self'.[10]

Visitors to the exhibition reflected upon this most recent history, up to the present day:

> It is about right about the system who let so many men and woman down. De-institutionalisation was the biggest balls up and the biggest mistake that happened in the western world where people had to leave the hospitals, people died on footpaths, in trains and bus shelters. Some people were taken back, some people used to fend for themselves, even their own families could not help them. They were sent to Mary Mac Hostel. The system now is a lot better, more services, more employment. But if they got it right in the first place they would not have the mess that they do now. Now the politicians and bureaucrats and the accountants do not know how to fix it.
>
> Male visitor aged 39

> Very thought provoking. Where do we house our mentally ill now . . . on the street?
>
> Female visitor aged 52[11]

MARGINAL COLLECTIONS

> The personal possessions, records etc make this exhibition a moving experience. The history is relevant—a sort of cycle that characterises all histories, but which *must* be recorded. GREAT.
>
> Male visitor aged 48[12]

With each shift in the ideology, form and practice of treatment at Goodna, the past was often destroyed or obscured. The material culture of the institution is patchy. Unlike other similar institutions in Australia and elsewhere, the hospital does not have a museum or organized historical collection. The remaining artefacts are a motley bunch, haphazardly saved and hoarded by staff and patients. An extensive collection of pharmaceutical items sits alongside institutional crockery in a display cabinet in a boardroom; a basement houses an array of historic furniture, medical equipment, craft objects, tools, books, phonograph records and other remnant items; while the corridors of another building are filled with striking works of art created by patients over the past decade or so. Most of the historical objects had no documentation; there was no knowledge about where they had come from, who had made them or when they had been used in the hospital. Sometimes it was not even known what these objects were.

The hospital also has an archive of medical records and patient casebooks. These records are not open to the public and access by researchers is strictly vetted—as curators of the exhibition, we were not allowed to view these records, for example. A broader archive can be located in a range of other local collections, such as the records of the Curator in Insanity, later Public Curator, at the Queensland State Archives. Here also are government publications and correspondence and a small number of photographic collections, produced mostly for Annual Reports. In short, the hospital's recognizable 'collections' of material culture did not offer a promising start for an exhibition. It was quickly apparent that other collections would need to be located and that these should be broadly conceived—a wide net had to be cast.

Unlike most museums, Museum of Brisbane itself does not have a substantial collection of historical artefacts and instead advocates for the use of community collections. Based on the premise that history is to be found throughout the city, not just in institutions and collections, and that the stories and objects of everyday people are vitally important to the history of the city, community collections lead and distinguish MoB's curatorial practice. We work with the community as both partners and participants in all our history exhibitions, collecting stories and borrowing items from individuals and groups. More than just an *ad hoc* adjunct to exhibitions, 'community collections' is an institutional ethos, a value that appreciates working with and for the broader community. Items in a community collection may be material objects, but may also include ideas and experiences, with or without any tangible evidence. In working with community collections, MoB taps into the city's collective memory in its many and various forms. This approach reaps rewards as previously unknown, rich and authentic content is located and fine-grained, emotional connections are created in the communal space of the museum. This is much more difficult to achieve if institutional collections are the only source of exhibition content.

In her chapter *Relating Collective Values*, Susan M. Pearce describes the dynamic system of collecting where at one end of a spectrum, the museum zone is a place of apotheosis where market and cultural values become one. The other end of the spectrum is the rubbish zone, where resides 'the unregarded detritus of commodity'. Community collections occupy the middle ground between these values—it is a 'messy, chancy, exciting place.'[13] Importantly, the process of using community collections recognises and assigns value to everyday and private objects, empowering them through a transformation from profane to sacred that occurs when an object becomes part of a collection, especially a museum collection. Community collections also reveal the emotional relationship between people and material objects, how objects come to embody and make tangible history and experience. In exhibitions, this relationship is then shared with visitors. With Remembering Goodna, existing collections were invigorated and new collections were generated or found through the community collections approach, leading to an exhibition that engaged museum visitors 'in a visceral and embodied journey through history.'[14]

SHARING COLLECTIONS

> I found it very moving while also glad to be learning about the history etc of Goodna. Left the City Hall a lot better person for having seen your well-researched exhibition. Thank you for your time and effort in putting this together and letting us, the people, share the story.
>
> Female visitor aged 63[15]

Working with community collections requires a shift in emphasis and approach from traditional curatorial work. Research is unlikely to take place in institutions; instead it is active and people-orientated. Curators need constantly to ask questions, to probe into people's lives, and uncover how objects come to stand in for experience. It is essential to establish relationships of trust so that people are able and willing to explore their memories safely and productively. Participants need to be supported and encouraged to recognize that their lives and collections have significance and that there is value in sharing these with the wider community. In the case of Remembering Goodna, there was much dangerous territory to be navigated. Many of the participants were vulnerable people whose personal history of institutionalistion had left them with few personal possessions but many painful memories. Drawing them into the process of creating an exhibition took sensitivity and creativity—new and different types of curatorial skills that are people-focused rather than object-focused. Empathy, or 'a kind of emotional literacy, an ability to work sensitively and astutely with the thoughts and feelings of others' is essential, as Kavanagh points out.[16]

The development of the exhibition was led by an interdisciplinary curatorium including medical staff, an advocate, a historian, a social worker and an arts worker, who worked together with museum staff to shape and guide the exhibition.[17] This group brought a great depth of experience and knowledge to the project, along with established relationships, personal connections and networks. Crucial also was the expertise—'emotional literacy'—from other fields such as social work, community development and psychology. The exhibition team also worked closely with past and present staff and patients of the hospital and their families, friends and advocates, tracked down through an intensive consultation period where these various communities were informed about the exhibition and invited to take part in its development. Only through meeting people who had lived and worked at the hospital could we really begin to grasp the nature of the place and develop an exhibition that would represent its history with authenticity, respect and dignity.

It is worthwhile re-visiting the aims of the exhibition as determined by the curatorium. In April 2007, these were stated as:

> To understand mental illness as a widely shared experience by exploring the perceptions and myths about mental illness and mental hospitals;
> To use the experiences and voices of patients to develop empathy in visitors to the exhibition;
> To acknowledge the complexity of mental illness—and its history of care, treatment and control;
> To create an experience of the institution as a place—the qualities of the landscape and buildings, relationship to Goodna village, the hospital as a workplace, visiting the hospital and so on.

These aims indicate how the exhibition was consciously intended as advocacy around the issue of mental ill health with the museum mindfully taking on a role as an agent of social change. To achieve this, the exhibition used a number of different presentation techniques, including both chronological and thematic approaches to the history; direct and largely unmediated recollections of patients, staff, families and advocates in the form of filmed interviews, audio stories, artworks, poetry and other writing; thematic groupings of images, documents, maps, stories and artefacts and an interactive map for exploring the history of the site and individual buildings.

Thematic groupings occupied the most physical space in the exhibition. The themes were: *'Going Up the Line'; Fences, Locks and Doors; Opening Doors; Labels; Birth, death and trauma; Speaking Up; Working Lives; Filling the Days; Breaking the Routine* and *Beyond Goodna*. These were supplemented with sets of evocative words, applied simply as outlines directly on to the walls, which deepened the feeling and emotion of the themes—another layer that then shaped how the filmed interviews were edited and presented within the thematic areas. The thematic groupings brought together extremely diverse material from across the institution's 150-year history and enabled multi-layered perspectives and diverse voices to emerge. Text and images were not presented together on integrated panels, instead each item was a separate, individual object that was then grouped with others in thematic 'clusters' on the wall so visitors could move from item to item and become absorbed in each one. 'Real' items such as letters, official documents, maps and photographs were individually reproduced while personal information, such as memoirs, poems and statements, was presented as pages in a journal, signaling to visitors that this was a first-person account.

Personal stories over a period of 150 years were extraordinarily difficult to track down. People who have lived in mental hospitals rarely leave much behind in the way of diaries, letters, or personal possessions, and as we were not able to access the hospital's records for the purpose

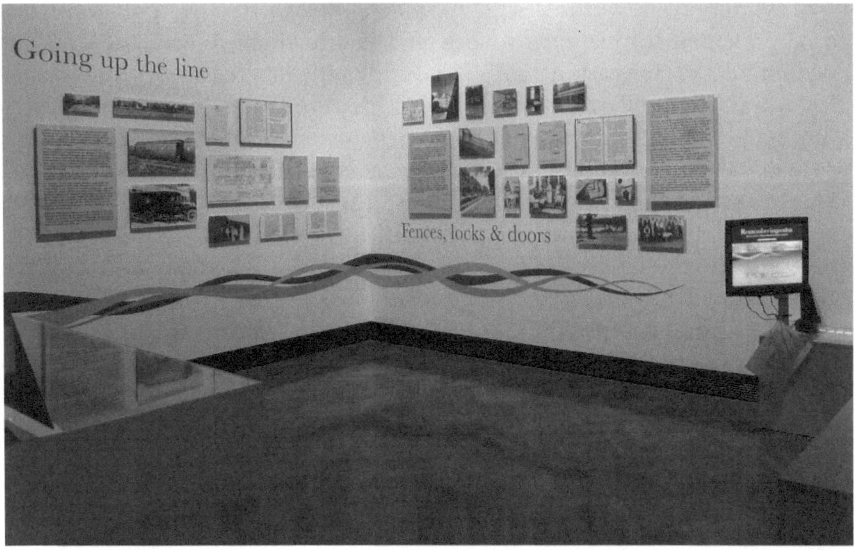

Figure 8.1 Thematic wall 'cluster', Remembering Goodna exhibition, Museum of Brisbane 2007–2008.
Source: Courtesy of Museum of Brisbane, Queensland, Australia.

of a public exhibition, every individual account we found was priceless. Our sources were often unlikely: an autobiography was found unexpectedly at a flea market; a psychiatrist's library donated to another local hospital had a personal diary in its midst; former staff members had kept poems and scraps of writing by patients and *Inside the Cuckoo's Nest,* a self-published book from 1977, proved to be a rich source of patients' stories.[18] Likewise, photographs—other than those officially sanctioned—were hard to locate. For most of the hospital's history, photography was forbidden on the hospital grounds and staff members were initially loath to admit that they had any images in their collections. As our relationships developed, however, a fascinating assortment of photographs materialised. A significant collection was also located in the holdings of the local Brisbane newspaper *The Courier-Mail.* Our good fortune here was that this collection was yet to become part of the centrally controlled system that required payment to access. We were able to use quite a number of these photographs, including rare images from the early 1950s. With such conditions of scarcity, we wanted every piece to be given due weighting in the exhibition design. In keeping with this egalitarian approach, the museum's didactic panels were presented as simply one item amongst these others. Artefacts were also arranged separately and thematically, placed on, and suspended above open plinths and accompanied by images and documents alongside personal stories and memories, again presented as journal pages.

Most importantly, this design approach allowed multiple points of view to be presented so that even fragmented and incomplete material could be accommodated. In working with personally remembered stories and memories, it was often the case that these conflicted. In the thematic clusters, they were simply placed side by side, allowing gaps and inconsistencies to have a place in the exhibition too. In some ways, it is easier to present an exhibition of the most arresting stories—the saddest, the most shocking or unexpected, the funniest and so on. It is much more difficult to capture the fine-grained, the everyday, the badly told and the offbeat and to balance these with the more dramatic. To do justice to Goodna's history and people's experiences there, we had to capture the contradictions: the place was isolated and self-contained yet also permeable and open; it was progressive at times but also conservative and shockingly retrograde at others. Individuals experienced the extremes of human existence; there was neglect and abuse, but tenderness and care as well. Ambiguity could never really be avoided entirely. The subtitle of the exhibition reflected this with our use of 'stories' rather than 'history'. Many among MoB's audience associate history with concepts of authority, progress and truth. Unlike 'history', 'stories' has a different set of associations. Stories are versions and there is room for inconsistency, lack of completeness and personal perspective. Everyone has a story to tell.

It was critical that the exhibition integrated the stories of the people who had lived and worked at the hospital and created opportunities for them to speak for themselves and give their versions of events. For many, the exhibition was their first chance to break the silences surrounding their experiences. Staff at the hospital had a strong collective identity that continued into retirement with regular reunion lunches and morning teas. Built around camaraderie and support at work, this group identity meant that few people found it possible to depart from well-worn narratives and express uncertainty about their time working at Goodna. The hospital's strict hierarchies reinforced these difficulties in speaking out. The exhibition provided an occasion for many to reveal lesser-known aspects of their working lives, to articulate fears and doubts but also to express their pride in prevailing in such a tough and demanding environment as well as the concern and affection they felt for many of the patients.

For former patients, involvement in the exhibition dredged up very difficult and painful memories, even re-traumatisation, and it was essential that they were supported throughout the process of remembering. Although participants told how hard it was to revisit the past, this seemed to be outweighed by the benefits they reported from sharing their experiences. They welcomed the opportunity to have their stories in the public realm, speaking to members of the wider community, not a specialised audience. As one participant commented: 'now [ordinary] people can see how we suffer with mental illness and how the environment was.'[19] The exhibition came some way in meeting a need for both private and communal commemoration. In bringing back the past, it allowed an opportunity for mourning in a context of public acknowledgement. In participating in the exhibition, many patients were aware that not only were they speaking for themselves but also for previous generations who were silenced in the historical record. For some, the exhibition was an important milestone in their personal journeys of recovery. 'I feel like I have crossed another bridge', said one former patient. 'I'm almost ready to close the book', said another.[20]

Community participation led to several major components in the exhibition and, in turn, generated rich new material to augment existing collections. In the first instance, MoB produced an eighty-minute documentary of interviews with past and present patients, past and present medical and non-medical staff, advocates, social workers, priests, friends and family members who all spoke frankly of their personal experiences of Goodna. The documentary was divided into twenty-minute segments, reflecting the exhibition's themes. Each segment was presented on a separate monitor attached to a bench that accommodated just two to three people. The stories were displayed in such a way that the person speaking was virtually life-size and the exchange between speaker and viewer was personal and close. However, mindful of the challenging and often distressing nature of the stories being told, the benches were designed so visitors sat with their backs against the wall so others couldn't watch over their shoulder and disturb the feeling of intimacy. Many visitors moved from bench to bench, watching all eighty minutes of stories.

A second component was effectively an 'exhibition within the exhibition'—the First Aid Box Project, curated by Neal Price, former psychiatric nurse, arts-worker and member of the curatorium. Standard metal first aid boxes were emptied of their medical contents, painted and decorated and filled instead with significant and meaningful items, both everyday and special objects that represented the ongoing process of recovery. People who currently live with mental health difficulties created the boxes and each conveyed a unique story. Several of the participants had spent time at Goodna. Visitors responded strongly to these very direct and yet symbolic representations of peoples' lives.

> Our favourite was the first aid boxes, they are very real and touching, even when you haven't been through what they have, you feel like you somehow know them, beautiful.
>
> Female visitors aged 16, 19 and 14

> A well-put together, very interesting exhibit. The first-aid boxes especially touched my heart, making me sad and hopeful all at the same time.
>
> Female visitor aged 25

> Very inspirational—the first aid boxes. Could relate to them and will start my own.
>
> Female visitor aged 20[21]

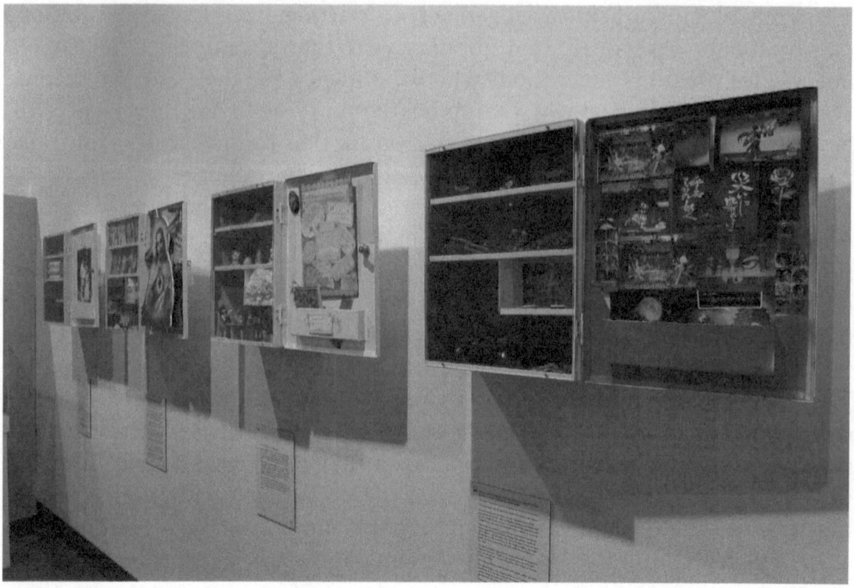

Figure 8.2 Installation view, First Aid Boxes Project, Remembering Goodna exhibition, Museum of Brisbane, 2007–2008.
Source: Courtesy of Museum of Brisbane, Queensland, Australia.

ENLIVENING COLLECTIONS

> Opens up the door to make you realise another side of things that everyday life seems to hide. Thank you so much for this; especially moving were the patients' stories. My kids were with me so we had a nice talk about this.
>
> Female visitor aged, 32[22]

One category of objects in the exhibition was the very ordinary, even generic objects that ostensibly had no special relationship to the history of a mental hospital. It was only in placing them in the museum, accompanied by stories from patients and staff that they took on particular significance. Take as an example the three huge aluminium teapots that were found amid the indiscriminate historical collection at the hospital. On first sight, they immediately conveyed life in an institution and the logistics of catering for large numbers of people. Then a staff member told us that the tea was known as 'Woogaroo brew' and that it came to the wards in these teapots with milk and sugar already mixed in, capturing a more powerful sense of institutional life. With this story, the denial of choice, the level of control over daily life and the disabling affects of never actually pouring a drink for yourself were able to be expressed in the exhibition. Likewise a galvanised iron food container that looked very much like an ordinary bucket provided another graphic illustration of the pragmatism and ugliness that characterised much of institutional life. Until the 1940s, meals were prepared in a large central kitchen and distributed to the wards in these containers, often arriving cold. Forty years of life in the institution were compressed by presenting the container alongside a 1985 article in the patient-produced hospital newsletter:

> One of the most important changes has taken place in the grounds of the hospital. Walking the roads and laneways now, one is no longer met with bins of unwanted foodstuffs, smelling strongly and in summertime commencing to putrefy . . . The containers containing the meals for patients used to be placed on the road awaiting conveyance to the wards by the busy staff. How different is the delivery of meals now! No sight of meals is seen. Food in neat containers is delivered straight to the kitchens or serveries.[23]

From a volume published privately by the hospital a poem by a patient, Beverley Stevenson, offered yet another viewpoint, using humour and absurdity to convey how patients coped with the boredom of institutional food and everyday life:

> This crazy place called Barrett E,
> So lost in space for all but me.
> I'm sitting here complacently,
> Just writing verse for all to see.
> Joan gets up and blows her stack,
> And for her there'll be no going back.
> Sylvia and Rosemary to name but a few,
> Are sick of eating only beef stew.
> Terry and mob with Anne and her gang
> Come daily to help me get over the pang.
> For Caramel Tarts and Cheesecake and cream,
> Now all I do is live a Midsummer Night's Dream. [24]

A visitor added another story:

> About thirty years ago I went to the kitchens at Goodna to deliver a parcel to one of the staff. A kitchen hand was putting pepper in all these cakes—they looked very nice. I asked him why he was doing this. He replied 'to get the dummies'.
>
> Male visitor aged 58[25]

This collection of items depicting the themes of institutional regimes and routines was rounded off with examples of the hospital-issue clothing that

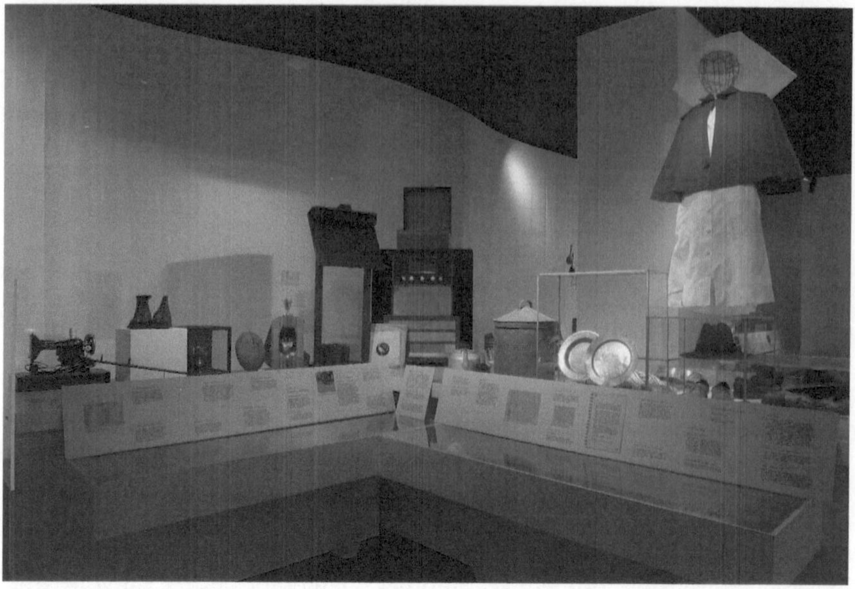

Figure 8.3 Thematic groupings of objects around everyday life in the institution, Remembering Goodna exhibition, Museum of Brisbane 2007–2008.
Source: Courtesy of Museum of Brisbane, Queensland, Australia.

patients were compelled to wear and a Government-issued clock, blanket and towel. Surprisingly, the towel is another forceful example of how an innocuous object can be powerfully transformed by memory. In the past, all Queensland hospitals used small white towels with 'Queensland Government' emblazoned in blue and they were certainly familiar to staff and patients at Goodna. Throughout the exhibition, these towels are referred to in a number of very dissimilar ways. A staff member who began his working life in the 1960s described his first day at work in one of the filmed documentaries. Almost like an initiation ritual, he was assigned to a large male ward, built in the 1920s, where about 170 men lived in very close confines. Many of the patients had schizophrenia, amongst a range of challenging conditions. He speaks about his fear and apprehension as he headed into the ward for the first time. On his way in, an 'old hand' with years of experience working at the hospital throws him a towel. He's confused and doesn't understand what it's for. Laughing, the old hand explains he'll need it to wipe the saliva off himself, as he needs to be prepared for patients to 'spit and slobber all over him'.

Patients recalled the towels differently:

> I have also witnessed bashings in the wards. I myself have had a wet towel placed around my neck and choked. On another occasion, a male staff member bashed my head against a wall, knocking skin off my

> face. He then said 'You won't do anything, you just hit your head on the wall.' Bashings are quite common in security wards. Staff bash patients for any reason they like. Some nurses used wet towels around patients' necks so as to choke them without leaving a mark.
> Larry, patient in 1968

> My most frightening memories are of a person called Billy who was in charge of so-called physical treatment. The procedure was to place a towel around one's neck and hit the person continually in the back. This happened to me on numerous occasions for simply asking a question or something equally trivial. He would tell the doctor I had attacked him and that was the reason for punishing me this way. This was not true but there was no point in denying his allegation because of my past record for assault. I think this treatment has resulted in a permanent back injury for my back now causes me quite a deal of discomfort.
> Sydney, patient in 1968[26]

These stories were displayed as journal pages in the thematic area *Birth, death and trauma*, while the staff member's story was in *Working lives* and the towel itself appeared in *Filling the days*. The stories were consciously scattered so that visitors could gradually gain a nuanced impression without conclusions being drawn for them. Some visitors' comments revealed a decisive response:

> It amazes me what human beings can subject their fellow human beings to if they feel them to be at some disadvantage.
> Male visitor aged 61

> I grew up in the suburb of Goodna, my family, my mum and dad, bought their first house there in 1970. We played football at a field near the hospital and would adventure up the Woogaroo Creek in our kayaks. Many of the fathers at the football club worked at the hospital, these were violent blokes who would drink to get drunk. As a kid I remember my parents sharing stories from these men, they were bastards.
> Male visitor aged 39

> Anyone is capable of cruelty—more so in a group. To think that institutions, which overlooked such misery, were actually sanctioned by law is very disturbing.
> Female visitor aged 63[27]

Another ordinary but also very affecting object on display was a long, leather coat owned by a police officer who was stationed in Rockhampton from 1935 to 1952. During this time, he wore the leather coat on many trips when he escorted patients destined for Goodna from Central Queensland.

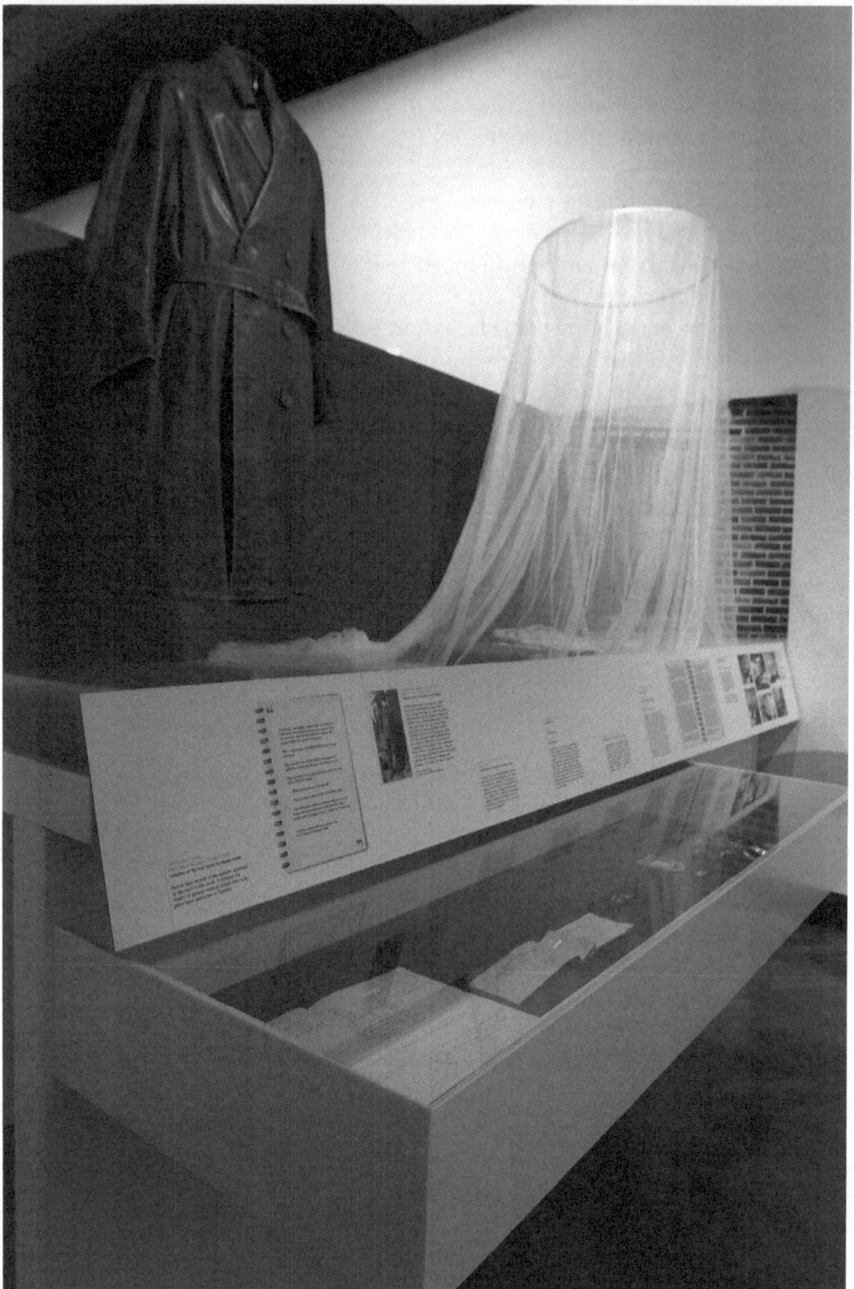

Figure 8.4 Installation detail showing police officer's coat, Remembering Goodna exhibition, Museum of Brisbane 2007–2008.
Source: Courtesy of Museum of Brisbane, Queensland, Australia.

Patients and their escorts spent the journey sitting up in the separate carriage designed specifically for the purpose of conveying 'lepers and lunatics'. We learned from the police officer's family that he felt a great deal of sympathy for the patients he accompanied. In an effort to keep appearances informal and to reduce patients' fear, police officers did not wear uniforms and this officer had the coat for warmth, conveying the discomfort of these trips. To highlight the long-standing dilemma of police involvement in this domain, the personal story of the coat was also supplemented with a quote from a letter of outrage from a local clergyman to the Colonial Secretary in 1869:

> Policemen, handcuffs, magistrates, horribly foul cells and a sense of criminality are only some of the miseries which frequently accompany the lunatic before he reaches Woogaroo. Why is the lunatic APPREHENDED on a charge of lunacy? Why should he be INDICTED for the severest affliction which can fall upon the human race? Why should he be consigned to the tender mercies of the POLICE court? . . . What crime has he committed? . . . The lunatic is taken INTO CUSTODY. Why? . . . the detention, with its corresponding horrors of police cell imprisonment is calculated to make a temporarily deranged man, a confirmed madman.[28]

A visitor echoed these sentiments and the compassion displayed by the officer who owned the coat:

> I remember in 1977 taking a man to Goodna hospital, I was twenty, a new policeman; he would have been forty-five and committed by his wife and a doctor. He seemed sad and confused that his wife would do that to him. He was disappointed to be taken in a police car, I felt he didn't deserve this treatment. The thought of it never left me!
>
> Male visitor aged 51[29]

Other artefacts in the exhibition were very specific and particular to the history of a mental hospital, highly potent and potentially distressing objects such as straitjackets, muffs, tranquilisers and other medications, Electroconvulsive Therapy (ECT) machines, keys for staff to operate taps, cigarette lighters kept chained to walls, and 'combinations'—the all-in-one, flannelette undergarments that female patients were forced to wear for many decades and which they couldn't undo for themselves. Personal stories and memories were used with these objects to humanise them and deter any potential voyeuristic intent on the part of visitors. Rather than just gaze upon a straightjacket, for instance, the stories encouraged visitors to imagine what it might be like to be inside one:

> Someone was screaming obscenities and the screaming sounded like a cornered animal. Then she realized that it was her voice and she was the animal cowering in a corner of the room, terrified and truly alone

> . . . one of them was holding a large canvas sheet and the doctor was standing in the doorway with the sheaf of papers still in his hand. And she was screaming through her tears. She was still crying when large male hands pulled her from her corner and laid her on the canvas sheet which had been spread on the trolley. And her tears became gasps for breath as the canvas sheet was wrapped around her and the leather straps that were attached to it were pulled across her legs and waist and chest and buckled tight. And, finally, she was silent as she realised that the only parts of her body that were free of the canvas were her head and her feet. And suddenly she wasn't cold any longer.
>
> . . . she was aware only of the brightness of the fluorescent lights that were set into the ceiling of the corridor of the hospital. She had never realised how bright fluorescent lights were before. The stark white lights were frightening in their intensity. The reality of what was happening was even more frightening. She cried softly as she lay, trussed in the strait-jacket. [30]

Responses from visitors indicated that this approach heightened their sensitivity to the plight of patients and also prompted them to critically reflect on the contemporary management of mental illness:

> It is a very moving and emotional experience. The displays are very well set out. It is sometimes necessary to expose the pain and suffering of those who are gone in order to see how far we have come in regards to the mental health system. We still have a long way to go.
>
> Male visitor aged 46[31]

CHANGING MINDS

The visitor comments woven throughout this chapter articulate how the wider Brisbane community received Remembering Goodna. More than just feedback or commentary, the richness of these contributions attest to the value of exhibitions in generating new collections and animating existing ones. The comments have now formed a new collection themselves, an added layer to a history already so intricate and nuanced. This new collection demonstrates how a dialogue was established between the museum's audience and the content of the exhibition, a dialogue that indicated a sincere, even profound, contemplation of the experience of mental ill health. Visitors became participants as an exchange of knowledge and experience took place in the space of the exhibition, even though their contribution was as uncomplicated as writing in a book. This exchange was complemented by public programs such as the *Sharing Lives,* a series of talks in which people living with mental health difficulties spoke openly about their experiences and museum visitors were invited to ask questions and share

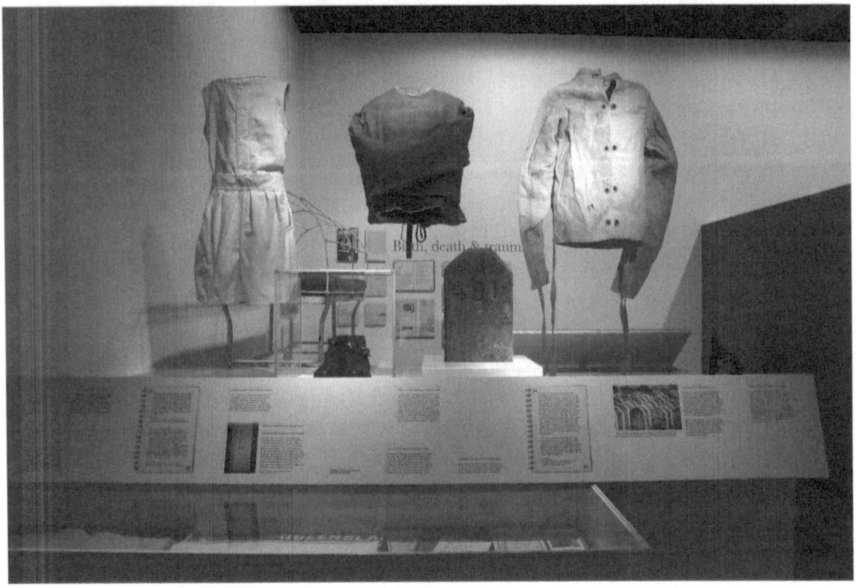

Figure 8.5 Straitjackets and combinations, Remembering Goodna exhibition, Museum of Brisbane 2007–2008.
Source: Courtesy of Museum of Brisbane, Queensland, Australia.

their own understanding of health and well-being. It was also underscored by the curatorial approach of presenting multi-faceted accounts of the institution's history, leaving visitors with questions rather than answers, and an invitation to contemplate these questions further in their own lives.

In using a community collections approach to developing the exhibition, the personal stories and memories of those who lived and worked at the hospital were able to permeate every part of the exhibition, conveying a complex and deeply-felt history. Remembering Goodna showed how community collections engage audiences, transform artifacts and express and represent historical experience in ways that conventional object-centred research approaches to exhibitions just cannot. Yet it can also been seen as a challenge to curatorial authority. In the case of Museum of Brisbane, community collections was already embedded as an approach; however, in many museums and similar institutions, this opening up of curatorial processes could pose ethical and practical difficulties. It requires a commitment to individuals that their memories and experiences will be treated with respect but also subject to institutional checks and balances, which must be negotiated carefully with participants throughout. Participants' expectations also need to be managed with honesty and openness. This takes time, which is often the scarcest commodity in the deadline-driven context of a temporary exhibition. Museums must also be willing to present difficult, open-ended, even contradictory, accounts of history; not take refuge in neat encapsulations. All of this can be deeply confronting for museum staff who may be grappling with their own personal responses to the subject matter as well as absorbing and processing the memories of participants. Working collaboratively with people with other skills, such as those represented in Remembering Goodna's curatorium, is one way to address these challenges. However, museums also need to acknowledge that this work brings ethical responsibilities that may need new skills and modified processes of engagement with both collections and communities.

Remembering Goodna showed that there are great benefits in collaborating with people whose lived experience has often been excluded from historical accounts. In applying the community collections approach to a subject as demanding and complex as how we understand and deal with mental illness, the exhibition also moved the museum visitor experience beyond that of curiosity or straightforward learning, into the realm of empathic transformation. Visitors expressed this best themselves:

> It's good to see how patients from Goodna see the outside world. I particularly feel sad and share some of their emotions. I think in our lives there is always some moment that we look back inside of our minds. It's just a human condition, if you're sick and sad or whatever you want to call it, that part of humans that make us what we are.
>
> Visitor, age not disclosed

> You really touched my soul!
>
> Female visitor aged 27[32]

NOTES

1. Gaynor Kavanagh, "Remembering Ourselves in the Work of Museums: Trauma and the Place of the Personal in the Public," in *Museums, Society, Inequality*, ed. Richard Sandell, Museum Meanings (London: Routledge, 2002), 111.
2. Museum of Brisbane (MoB) is a city museum that explores the history and contemporary cultures of Brisbane, the capital city of Queensland. It operates as part of the Brisbane City Council and is located in City Hall. 60,000 people visited the Remembering Goodna exhibition over a four and a half month period.
3. Visitors were invited to respond to the exhibition and/or to contribute their own stories or personal experiences of the mental hospital; 640 substantial written comments were left and included the visitors' name, gender, age and place of residence.
4. This slogan came into use by disability activists in the 1990s; its origins are unclear, it is the title of a book by James I. Charlton, *Nothing About Us Without Us: Disability Oppression and Empowerment* (Berkeley: University of California Press),1998.
5. Museum of Brisbane, Visitors' Comments, Remembering Goodna exhibition (Brisbane, 2007–2008).

6. Mark Finnane, "Wolston Park Hospital 1865–2001: A Retrospect, *Queensland Review* 15, no. 2, (2008): 39–58"; Raymond Evans, "Charitable Institutions of the Queensland Government to 1919" (MA Thesis, University of Queensland, 1970); Catharine Coleborne and Dolly MacKinnon, eds., *Madness in Australia: Histories, Heritage and the Asylum* (St Lucia: University of Queensland Press, 2003).
7. For other studies of these familiar themes see Stephen Garton, *Medicine and Madness: A Social History of Insanity in New South Wales 1880–1940* (Kensington, NSW: University of New South Wales Press, 1988); M. J. Lewis, *Managing Madness: Psychiatry and Society in Australia 1788–1980* (Canberra: Australian Government Publishing Service, 1988); Coleborne and MacKinnon, *Madness in Australia*; Warwick Brunton, "The Origins of Deinstitutionalisation in New Zealand," *Health and History* 5, no. 2 (2003): 75–103; Dolly Mackinnon and Catharine Coleborne, "Introduction: Deinstitutionalisation in Australia and New Zealand," *Health and History,* 1–17.
8. On the function of labour in the Wolston Park hospital see Mark Finnane, "The Ruly and the Unruly: The Uses of Isolation in the Management of the Insane," in *Isolation: Places and Practices of Exclusion*, ed. Alison Bashford and Carolyn Strange, Routledge Studies in Modern History (London: Routledge, 2003), 89–103.
9. For a comparison of Australian hospitals at this time see Alan Stoller, *Report on Mental Health Facilities and Needs of Australia* (Canberra, 1955).
10. Museum of Brisbane, filmed interview with former patient Stephen Morgan, Remembering Goodna exhibition (Brisbane, 2007–2008). For a comprehensive study of these changes from institutional and public policy perspectives see Darrel Phillip Doessel, "A Historical Perspective on Mental Health Services in Australia: 1883–84 to 2003–04," *Australian Economic History Review* 49, no. 2 (July 2009): 173–197; D. P. Doessel and others, "Deinstitutionalisation and Managerialism in Queensland's Public Psychiatric Institutions: Challenging 'Rhetoric' with Empirical Results," *Australian Journal of Public Administration* 68, no. 4 (December 2009): 459–483; and from a social history perspective see Brunton, "The Origins of Deinstitutionalisation in New Zealand," *Health and History* 5, no. 2 (2003): 75–103; Finnane, "Opening Up and Closing Down: Notes on the End of an Asylum," *Health and History* 11, no. 1 (2009): 9–24; Stephen Garton, "Seeking Refuge: Why Asylum Facilities Might Still be Relevant for Mental Health Care Services Today," *Health and History* 11, no. 1 (2009): 25–45.
11. Museum of Brisbane, Visitors' Comments, Remembering Goodna exhibition (Brisbane, 2007–2008).
12. Ibid.
13. Susan M. Pearce, *On Collecting. An Investigation into Collecting in the European Tradition*, Collecting Cultures (London: Routledge, 1995), 396.
14. Fiona Paisley, "Peeling Back History: The Remembering Goodna Exhibition," *Health and History* 11, no. 1 (2009): 174.
15. Museum of Brisbane, Visitors' Comments, Remembering Goodna exhibition (Brisbane, 2007–2008).
16. Kavanagh, "Remembering Ourselves," 111.
17. The exhibition had its origins in a research project, led by historian Mark Finnane of Griffith University and funded by the Australian Research Council, which subsequently evolved as a partnership between the university, Museum of Brisbane and The Park Centre for Mental Health. The curatorium comprised Nadia Beer, Jo Besley, Mark Finnane, Deborah Gilroy, Leanne Kelly, Carol Low and Neal Price.

18. Jim Gardner, *Inside the Cuckoo's Nest: Madness in Australia* (Brisbane: Planet Publishing, 1977).
19. Interview between Joanna Besley and former patient who shared her story on film in the exhibition, March 2008.
20. Ibid.
21. Museum of Brisbane, Visitors' Comments, Remembering Goodna exhibition (Brisbane, 2007–2008).
22. Ibid.
23. *The Colony Times* (Brisbane), 1985.
24. Patients at Wolston Park Hospital, *In Dark Hours* (Brisbane: Wolston Park Hospital, 1997), 22.
25. Museum of Brisbane, Visitors' Comments, Remembering Goodna exhibition (Brisbane, 2007–2008).
26. Gardner, *Inside the Cuckoo's Nest*, 27.
27. Museum of Brisbane, Visitors' Comments, Remembering Goodna exhibition (Brisbane, 2007–2008).
28. Correspondence, Reverend Draper to Colonial Secretary, 16 January, 1869, quoted in Evans, Raymond, "Charitable Institutions of the Queensland Government to 1919" (M.A. Thesis, University of Queensland, 1970), 57.
29. Museum of Brisbane, Visitors' Comments, Remembering Goodna exhibition (Brisbane, 2007–2008).
30. June Wrigley, recounting being put in a straitjacket in 1965 [at Goodna], from her memoir *The Less Travelled Way* (Melbourne: Collins Dove, 1990), 42.
31. Museum of Brisbane, Visitors' Comments, Remembering Goodna exhibition (Brisbane, 2007–2008).
32. Ibid.

Part III

Bodies and Fragments

9 In the Interests of Science
Gathering Corpses from Lunatic Asylums

Helen MacDonald

INTRODUCTION

Lunatic asylum mortuaries were busy places during the nineteenth century, inside which several different kinds of post-mortem work were carried out. Autopsies were undertaken when a coroner ordered one, in order to determine the cause of a person's death. In addition, post-mortem examinations were performed when an asylum medical officer sought inside a particular body for signs of its morbid anatomy. During both of these kinds of examinations, body parts were routinely removed and retained as specimens and to be turned into preparations for museums. There, they joined material removed from corpses that had been dissected by students in medical schools. Those bodies had been collected from institutions including lunatic asylums, under the terms of Anatomy Acts in Britain and Australia, joining corpses taken from workhouses, hospitals and gaols. All were conscripted as subjects for dissection.

THE LAW AND ANATOMICAL EXAMINATIONS

Until 1832, medical schools in England and Scotland obtained corpses for their students in nefarious ways. The only lawful supply was a small one that came from the gallows when murderers received the secondary punishment of being dissected.[1] Other bodies were therefore purchased from grave robbers or imported from Ireland and France, while medical men who held hospital appointments obtained the bodies of patients who had died in their care. Then, in 1828, it was discovered that in Edinburgh two men, William Burke and William Hare, had murdered sixteen people in order to sell their bodies to an anatomist, and three years later anatomy murderers were also discovered operating in London.[2]

This was the context in which British parliamentarians developed *An Act for Regulating Schools of Anatomy* (1832), a contentious statute that gave unspecified officials 'lawful possession' of bodies for the purpose of enabling them to send these to medical schools rather than directly burying them.[3] No institutions were designated in the Act, but their identity was clear to those who followed the parliamentary debates over 1831–1832. Henceforth, officials in positions of authority in British workhouses, hospitals and gaols were authorised to send corpses to medical schools.

Two caveats applied. People could leave a formal, witnessed protest against an 'anatomical examination' or dissection being performed on their bodies; and relatives could claim corpses for burial (within 48 hours of the death) and so remove them from the institution's dead house. The Act's boosters asserted that this meant that only 'unclaimed' bodies would be sent to schools: those of people who had no relatives whose feelings would be harmed by knowing that the body had been mutilated. However the Anatomy Act did not require officials to notify either residents or their relatives of this law's existence, nor of their ability to dissent to a dissection. In addition, because British medical schools urgently needed corpses consideration for relatives' views was undercut. As the Duke of Sussex articulated this in the House of Lords, while

> no man can more earnestly desire than I do that the delicacy of family feeling should not be outraged . . . if some arrangements be not speedily made, you will drive the study of anatomy altogether from this country.[4]

The larger good of medical education required that the greatest possible number of bodies was made available to students, and the institutions in which numerous people lived and died in industrialising Britain made ideal places to collect them.

Inspectors of Anatomy were appointed under this statute, and the letter books that they kept for the rest of the century reveal how difficult it proved to be for people to extricate themselves and their relatives from becoming subjects for dissection. The right to dissent from post-mortem use of remains was routinely subverted and the inspectors themselves were complicit in this.[5] In addition the law only dealt with entire corpses, having neglected to provide for the removal and retention of body parts.[6] Yet this activity was frequently performed in medical schools, of which anatomical museums were an important part; and specimens, as Jonathan Reinarz has pointed out, were easier to update from the bodies of the sick poor than were the books in medical schools' libraries.[7] Indeed, so little of a dissected corpse might finally be sent to a burial ground that, to disguise this lack, coffins were weighed down with debris; 'so mixed', in Inspector John Bacot's words, 'with extraneous matter' as to cause outrage should the coffin be opened and its contents inspected.[8]

Where whole bodies were concerned, the legislation had given the anatomy inspectors no role in finding these for the schools, but they quickly assumed this additional responsibility, for supplies remained scarce. The inspectors constantly wrote to beguile institutions to 'co-operate with the

Act', pointing out as an enticement how much money a parish or institution could save by disposing of corpses in this way rather than burying them. The extent to which an institution's officials could go in turning corpses to profitable use came to public attention in a dramatic way in 1857–8, during a scandal at the St Mary Newington Workhouse in Surrey. It resulted in an important test case of the Anatomy Act, *R v Feist* (1858), heard in London's Central Criminal Court. Workhouse master Alfred Feist, in league with the parish undertaker, had been selling corpses to Guy's Hospital medical school and disguising that fact by organising sham funerals for inmates' relatives to attend. This case established that workhouse masters had legal possession of corpses under the Anatomy Act, and Feist was therefore found not guilty of contravening it. As the solicitors who had prosecuted the case on behalf of the St Mary Newington parish subsequently pointed out, the case had also established that under the Anatomy Act neither inmates nor relatives needed to be alerted to the existence of this law.[9]

GATHERING ASYLUM BODIES

No mention had been made of lunatic asylums as sources of corpse supply during the parliamentary debates surrounding the Anatomy Act. During the first three decades of its operation these institutions contributed a small number of corpses to medical schools. However from the 1850s that changed, to such an extent that by 1914 lunatic asylums were sending nearly as many bodies to be dissected as were the Poor Law establishments upon which the Act had, in the main, relied. Of the 275 bodies received in London's schools in 1913–1914, 153 had arrived from Poor Law infirmaries, 117 from the metropolitan asylums board and county council asylums, and five from general hospitals.[10]

The legislation had a distinctively hard edge where lunatic asylums were concerned. At least on paper, the anatomy statute enabled workhouse residents and general hospital patients, should they know of the Act, to make a rational choice about whether or not they wished to be dissected when they died. However people were confined in lunatic asylums because they were deemed to be incapable of making rational decisions. As Reverend John Burden wrote in 1867 to the Medical Superintendent of the Gloucester Lunatic Asylum:

> Insanity is a misfortune, not a crime and though it may be fair enough to dissect the bodies of those who have undergone the extreme penalty of the law, or who die in Jail or even commonly of those who have died in public hospitals, to which they have sought access voluntarily, yet surely in asylums, where the insane poor are detained (without any consent of their own or friends) the practise [*sic*] ought not to be permitted.[11]

Two of Burden's parishioners had approached him to act on their behalf with this asylum, after they had arrived there to view their father's corpse and found that it had been cut open in the asylum mortuary. This appears to have been a case of the medical superintendent performing a post-mortem examination of the body and then disguising his work beneath the shroud and cap in which the corpse was dressed. But Burden suspected that the body had been dissected because his parishioners, too poor to pay for a private funeral, had taken up the asylum's offer to bury their father. Did this mean, Burden demanded to know, that the asylum considered that the man's daughters had effectively *sold* the body to the asylum?

While *R v Feist* had established in law that workhouse masters were in lawful possession of inmates' corpses, no case had clarified who was in an equivalent position with regard to asylum bodies. Several asylum Committees of Visitors sought to determine the legal status of activities inside these mortuaries—both the post-mortem examinations that were performed there, and the collection of bodies for medical schools. The Littlemore Asylum's visitors wrote to ask the Commissioners in Lunacy to obtain the Crown Law Officer's opinion on the matter of precisely who was in lawful possession of bodies in their asylum, and whether an asylum medical officer had 'the strict legal right' to perform post-mortems. The Commissioners responded that neither the visitors nor asylum medical officers were empowered by law to cause post-mortems to be made.[12]

In this absence of clarity around whether or not asylum authorities were in lawful possession of the dead for the Anatomy Act's purpose, provincial medical schools assumed that they were, and set about the work of obtaining these bodies. They made private arrangements with local asylums: the Wakefield Lunatic Asylum supplied the Leeds medical school; the Hull Borough Asylum sent corpses to its local school.[13] And they also used the anatomy inspectors to bring other asylums into the fold. Working on the schools' behalf, the inspectors approached individual medical men who were connected with lunatic asylums, knowing that such men would understand better than lay people did, that the schools' great want of corpses must be satisfied lest illegalities follow. Thus the anatomy inspector wrote collegially to Dr D. F. Tyerman at Colney Hatch Lunatic Asylum in 1857 to ask for his assistance with regard to obtaining that institution's unclaimed bodies, closing his letter in the following way: 'as a member of our profession I cannot doubt your readiness to forward my views.'[14]

This chapter is primarily concerned with the collection of bodies from lunatic asylums for use in medical schools, rather than with asylum-based post-mortem examinations. However, during both dissections and such autopsies interesting parts were habitually excised from bodies for closer inspection and/or collected for museums. From the many post-mortems Dr Robert Boyd performed in the Somerset County Lunatic Asylum, he examined 528 brains.[15] When James Crichton-Browne at the West Riding Lunatic Asylum in Wakefield, Yorkshire left this asylum in 1876 to become Lord

Chancellor's Visitor in Lunacy, he regretted that the move cut his research short. At that time his sample of brains ('Removed from the skull by a pathologist—and never by a porter'), collected over three years, comprised those of 244 men and 156 women.[16] And the founding medical superintendent (from 1851) at the Wiltshire County Asylum for pauper lunatics, Dr John Thurnam, collected pathological specimens which he later donated to the Hunterian Museum at the Royal College of Surgeons in London.[17] As will be discussed later in this chapter, Thurnam also had wider interests in human remains. Together with Dr Joseph Barnard Davis, England's premier skull collector, he disinterred ancient bones from barrows, which the two men catalogued in a book titled *Crania Britannica, Delineations and Descriptions of the Skulls of the Aboriginal and Early Inhabitants of the British Islands* (1856–1865).[18] At Thurnam's invitation, on 18 March 1860 Davis visited the Wiltshire Asylum, pencilling in his notebook that the 200 or so lunatics he observed there were 'remarkable for large faces . . . heads are large & differ much in form . . . very large noses are common.'[19] Davis, as another of his fellow collectors later recalled, looked at the heads of the living 'simply as potential skulls.'[20]

Where subjects for dissection were concerned, provincial British medical schools had particular difficulties in finding workhouses with sufficient corpses to satisfy their needs and in this context turned to lunatic asylums. The schools worked with the anatomy inspectors, government officials and asylum visitors in this regard. In 1864 provincial anatomy inspector Dr George Cursham tried to persuade the Cambridgeshire Lunatic Asylum's visitors to send their unclaimed dead to the Cambridge University medical school, and sought the assistance of the Commissioners in Lunacy.[21] However the Commissioners proved to be wily operators. They had no desire for any acquiescence at the removal of corpses on their part to come to public notice, and so refused to approve it, fearing that this would increase the 'prejudice' against sending people to lunatic asylums.[22] The Cambridge medical school interpreted this as 'unfavourable, not absolutely prohibitory but dissuasive' advice. Professor of Anatomy Dr Humphry set to work behind the scenes, travelling to London to speak personally with the Commissioners, without avail.[23]

Thirteen years later Humphry approached the visitors of the St Nect Asylum, which subsequently resolved that 'subject to the previous examination by the medical Superintendent of this Asylum in all cases required by him for that purpose' they would send the corpses of all dead patients who were unclaimed and had no known friends to the university's school of medicine for 'Anatomical Purposes'.[24] Once again, when the Commissioners in Lunacy were approached they ambiguously responded that they had 'no power to interfere in the arrangements the Visitors may see fit to adopt with regard to the unclaimed bodies of patients dying in the Three Counties Asylum', and feared 'that the proposed regulation if it becomes notorious, might produce a prejudice against the asylum in the minds both of the patient and of the poor generally' and thus interfere with the institution's 'usefulness'.[25] When Alexander Macalister became Professor of Anatomy at Downing College in Cambridge he re-energised the quest for corpses there, writing a circular in 1884 in which he offered to pay such expenses as railway carriage from institutions—including asylums—to the school, together with other expenses.[26]

In 1899 the Cambridgeshire Asylum visitors again attempted to make a rule enabling them to supply the Cambridge school, and once more the Commissioners in Lunacy refused to endorse it.[27] Anatomy Inspector Thomas Pickering Pick wrote on the university's behalf to assure the Home Office that such corpse removal would be accomplished stealthily. 'Every care would be taken to remove the bodies decently and without the cognisance of any one beyond the officials of the Institution from which they are removed'.[28] This was the secretive way in which the Anatomy Act worked across the course of the nineteenth century. Stealth was promoted by successive anatomy inspectors and condoned by government officials and parliamentarians.

REGIONAL DISTINCTIONS

Important differences existed in the practices that arose under this legislation within the British Isles, including with regard to lunatic asylums. Ina Scherder's research is revealing that in Ireland, lunatic asylums were a compliant source of corpses for medical schools.[29] In 1884, questions about this were raised in the House of Commons when the Lord Lieutenant of Ireland was asked about the connection between the Cork District Lunatic Asylum and Queen's College, Cork. Member of parliament Mr Healy sought in vain from Chief Secretary Trevelyan the precise number of asylum bodies that had been disposed of in this way. But, using the time-honoured method employed by governments to deflect discussion of the Anatomy Act, Trevelyan first insisted that there was nothing wrong with the arrangement since only 'unclaimed' bodies would be so used, since the asylum's 'rules' would ensure that relatives were informed of other deaths, and that the law was being 'fully complied with at Cork'. Then Trevelyan closed the conversation by insisting it was an unseemly one for public debate. He asked Healy not to 'press his inquiries' in the House, for they involved details that should not be given in Parliament. This brought a halt to Healy's enquiries, though he closed them by pointing out for the benefit of the Hansard recording that the Chief Secretary had 'declined to say whether the bodies of these unfortunate deceased Irish lunatics were given over for dissection' and this indicated to him that Trevelyan 'considered such a practice scandalous.'[30]

Elsewhere, I have shown how Scotland's anatomy inspectors had become integrated into the system of corpse procurement over the course of the nineteenth century—in a way that England's medical schools could only envy. This was due in no small part to the ongoing salience of Edinburgh's infamous Burke and Hare murders which, it was believed, made Scottish people's abhorrence of the medical schools particularly strong. One early consequence had been that north of the border, town and city authorities provided the schools with a level of direct support that was not the case in England. By the late 1830s a system of 'funeratories' was being established through which to secretly supply medical schools with corpses. These places appeared to be no more than town dead-houses, convenient sites to lodge bodies prior to their burial. But they had actually been established at the behest of Edinburgh's anatomy teachers as sites from which they could obtain bodies without appearing to do so, given that Edinburgh's poor houses were reluctant to be seen to be complying with the Anatomy Act.[31]

English medical men desired such a system to be replicated south of the border. As was argued in a petition to the House of Commons in 1841, it was often difficult to define who was 'the lawful possessor' of a body and the Anatomy Act should be amended to compel such men to send corpses to the schools, for as matters stood such 'public functionaries' universally feared to exercise this right. The petitioners argued that a new clause should be inserted into the legislation to provide for 'the immediate removal of unclaimed bodies to a public dead-house, whence they may be removed, whether to the burial-ground or dissection room, without public observation.'[32] In other words, the Scottish funeratory system should be replicated in England.

By the end of the nineteenth century Scotland's anatomy inspectors had become pivotal to the way that the funeratories worked. Inspector (Dr) James Russell held, in addition to this role, those of chairman and treasurer of Edinburgh's association of anatomy lecturers (which paid the wages of funeratory staff).[33] The minutes of that association's meetings were being recorded in Inspector Russell's letter book. Having Russell as Scotland's anatomy inspector also suited teachers there for other reasons. He had learned his anatomy from Professor William Turner at the University of Edinburgh's medical school, and had also been Turner's anatomy demonstrator, in grand new apartments whose facilities were 'unsurpassed in the British Empire.' [34] These were grouped around a large new anatomical museum which was filled with specimens of which Turner was particularly proud. It would come to house an extraordinarily large collection of body parts that illustrated all kinds of anatomy—normal, pathological and anthropological. Professor Richard Berry, another Turner-trained man, noted that Turner 'was not partial to models', preferring dead bodies to these.[35]

To obtain his bodies, Turner worked closely with Inspector Russell to open up Scotland's institutions, including lunatic asylums, as sources of corpses. The two men found some asylum officials were reluctant to comply. The medical superintendent at Rosewell Asylum, Dr R.W. Cameron, refused on the grounds that there was

> Such a feeling of repugnance in the public mind to any method of disposal of bodies other than the ordinary burial that I hesitate to do anything that might lay my actions open to misconstruction or give rise to any vulgar superstitions.[36]

Dr Campbell of the Perth District Asylum argued that unclaimed asylum bodies did not belong to the inspector of anatomy, but rather to the inspector of the poor of the parish to which the deceased person was chargeable.[37] However with other asylums, Turner and Russell had more success. On June 2, 1882 the two men visited Dr James Rutherford, physician-superintendent of the Barony Parochial Asylum for Insane at Lenzie, a pauper establishment close to Glasgow which housed more than four hundred patients.[38] Rutherford agreed to send corpses into the system, though he soon had cause to complain when Russell's clerk (who was also a funeratory employee) arrived at the asylum to collect a body at an improper hour and in a conveyance that was far from 'decent looking'.[39]

This asylum's board of governors was unaware of the deal their superintendent had struck with Russell and Turner. When Rutherford left the Barony Parochial Asylum, Professor of Anatomy John Cleland at Glasgow University warned Russell not to approach the board, and asked him if the schools could instead 'draw on' the Barony asylum's corpses without alerting its members.[40] Meanwhile Rutherford, who had taken up a position at the Crichton Royal Institute in Dumfries, secretly continued to supply bodies to schools from there. In 1887 he sent Turner a corpse even though the local parish had instructed him to instead bury it. Rutherford wrote to inform Inspector Russell that—to disguise his donation—he had charged the parish for a coffin and a burial as if the body had not been sent to a school.[41]

Such secrecy was required even though local laws in Edinburgh and Glasgow had effectively made it compulsory for Scottish institutions to comply with the Anatomy Act. Russell and Turner had negotiated with Scotland's Lord Advocate to add a clause to the Police and Health Bills which specified that the bodies of all people who died without known relatives should be removed, disinfected and buried 'according to the provisions' of the Anatomy Act.[42] That is, they should be dissected. Inspector Russell had also written to Professor Cleland at Glasgow University to ask him and his ballies (magistrates) to influence local members of parliament to give this clause a 'silent reception'.[43] Cleland readily agreed, later writing to warn Russell that no one must imagine that the Burgh Police and Health Scotland Bill went near 'anatomical matters'.[44] Once the Bills passed, Professor George Macleod in Glasgow believed that he would be in a much stronger position in again approaching the Barony asylum board.[45] Russell had found that making 'private explanations' of the situation to its members was the best method of gaining the results he required:

> I have a strong feeling that private explanations of the Anatomy Act to members of the Board is the method most in accordance with the spirit of the Act and that the public have a right to expect that the discussion and arrangements connected with disagreeable subjects such as Anatomy should be conducted as far as possible in private.[46]

From April 1889 the Barony Parish supply of bodies significantly increased.[47] In their quest for bodies, Turner's successors at the University of Edinburgh—Professor Daniel Cunningham, followed by Professor Arthur Robinson—were as relentless as he had been. Robinson worked through asylum officials in ways that further reveal how such matters were organised. He found a supportive asylum official in the form of Dr Robert Campbell at the Stirling District Asylum, and sent the man a supply of syringes and instructions on how to inject bodies to ensure that they were well preserved and so arrived in the University of Edinburgh's dissecting room in optimum condition. Campbell subsequently worked at the Stirling asylum as if he was Robinson's dissecting-room assistant. In its mortuary he injected bodies 'towards the heart along the radial artery' through a pipe that he had inserted into the artery in the ordinary pulse region. For this, he made up solutions following Robinson's recipes and used these according to the state of each particular corpse, and when the school would require it. If the body was not to be dissected immediately, a mixture of twenty ounces of Formol and sixty of methylated spirits would be required—unless the body was 'spare and not moist' (for then water could replace the methylated spirit). If the corpse only needed to last for a week, less solution was required: for a 'small spare body' only twenty ounces, but thirty ounces if the body was large. Water need only be added to the Formol if the body was 'thin and dry'; methylated spirits if it was 'fat or sloppy'.[48]

'EXAMINING' CORPSES

Asylum bodies were frequently subjected to post-mortem examinations in these institutions' mortuaries, on the rationale that only by this means could the actual cause of the person's death be established and foul play ruled out. Though family members who learned of such examinations protested about them, the Commissioners in Lunacy considered that to prohibit these post-mortems would be 'highly inexpedient' and lead to improper care and treatment of pauper lunatics.[49]

However, the medical schools which sought corpses from lunatic asylums had no wish to receive bodies that had already been subjected to a post-mortem.[50] Professor Robinson emphasised to Dr Campbell at the Stirling asylum that the bodies he sent to the University of Edinburgh should arrive there intact. This was a contentious instruction, as men at the Stirling asylum were aware of the kind of cruelties towards patients that could occur. Dr George Robertson wrote in 1902 of his experiences there, where abusive practices had been 'inherited from the past' and were 'difficult to eradicate'. A 'great deal of unnecessary force or roughness, not amounting to actual violence' was employed and sometimes, albeit rarely, culminated in deaths. In Robertson's view these were 'a blessing in disguise', for traces of the assaults then became visible to medical authorities and offenders were punished. However Robertson also knew that violence in lunatic asylums was rarely reported. One attendant whom he had questioned at Stirling told him of witnessing many abuses which he had failed to report, knowing that if he did so he 'would not have had the life of a dog' with the other attendants.[51]

Still, the University of Edinburgh medical school did not wish to receive bodies that had been opened in asylum mortuaries. Professor Arthur Robinson therefore negotiated with the General Board of Control for Scotland to avoid post-mortems being carried out on 'unclaimed' asylum corpses—though arguably these were the very deaths that most needed to be investigated, people who had died without relatives or friends to visit them. Robinson sought the Board's approval for the bodies of people who died 'alone' in asylums to be sent to the University of Edinburgh's medical school intact, in the higher interests of his students' medical education. To this the Board agreed, urging the 'great importance of a *Post-mortem* examination being made of every patient who dies in an asylum whenever the consent of relatives or others empowered to give it can be obtained' both in the interests of science and to reassure the living that these deaths were due to natural causes. But when there were no friends or relatives, the Board instructed that the corpse could be sent to be dissected instead.[52] Professor Robinson subsequently wrote to Dr Campbell at the Stirling District Asylum '[u]nder these circumstances we shall be very glad if you let us have as many bodies as possible of those you are able to send without making a post mortem.' He understood that in some cases Campbell would prefer to autopsy a corpse at the asylum, but assured him that if he chose not to do that, the medical school would take care to note, during the dissection, anything that was 'abnormal' and to pay 'attention to any particular point to which you draw our notice.' Thus, while Campbell worked on the university's behalf by injecting bodies for their students to dissect, Robinson promised to work on the asylum's behalf by noticing abnormalities in particular corpses. Then Robinson reassured Campbell that when asylum residents died alone, the Commissioners of the Board of Control would accept as sufficient reason for no post-mortem being performed, an annotation on the Notice of Death that the body had been sent to an anatomical school 'for examination there'.[53]

A dissection was different to a post-mortem examination. It was performed by medical students, in a place far removed from the site and context of the person's death. Nevertheless, Dr Campbell informed Robinson that he understood his desire for intact bodies and reassured him that he could 'rest assured that I will see that your desire is complied with in all cases except where there is an absolute necessity for the *post mortem*'.[54]

And Robinson also sought bodies from further afield. He maintained his predecessor William Turner's connections with former Edinburgh students who now lived in the Antipodes, notably Dr William Ramsay Smith in Adelaide, South Australia. On 7 March 1911 Robertson wrote to Smith in the following terms: 'I need scarcely say, as custodian of the Museum, how very much I am indebted to you for the last and previous consignments nor how gladly I shall receive any other specimens you send.'[55]

A WORLD AWAY

The English and Scottish ways of procuring corpses for medical students was part of the cultural baggage brought by British-trained medical men to the Australian colonies. There, they taught in medical schools, took up positions in hospitals and lunatic asylums, and acted as anatomy inspectors under legislation that had taken the British Anatomy Act of 1832 as its model and added some colonial distinctions.[56] There were no workhouses in Australia, so instead the primary sources of corpses there were hospitals, together with asylums of one kind or another—destitute, lunatic, immigrant.[57]

One important difference in the Australian statutes was that these reduced the time during which relatives could claim corpses for burial, from the forty-eight hours allowed in Britain to a mere twelve.[58] The effect this would have had not escaped parliamentarians as these Bills were being debated. It became a point of contention in New South Wales in 1881 when parliamentarian and lawyer William Foster argued that enabling 'any person who was in lawful possession of a body' to give it up for dissection unless relatives 'happened to be near at hand to object' was something that would 'never be tolerated in any civilised community.'[59]

A second difference in Australia was that two colonial statutes specified the places from which bodies could be obtained, following the example set by the 1875 New Zealand anatomy statute.[60] As Dolly MacKinnon has shown, in Victoria this was achieved through an 1876 amendment to the Medical Practitioners' Act that named hospitals, lunatic asylums and gaols.[61] In South Australia, *An Act to Authorize the Establishment of Schools of Anatomy and to Regulate the Practice of Anatomy Therein, 1884* enabled the Chief Secretary to authorise in that colony:

> . . . the medical officer of any public institution, supported wholly or in part by funds from the general revenue, to permit the body of a person who dies in such institution (unless it is a public hospital) to undergo anatomical examination in any school of anatomy or in any public institution [.]

Hospitals had only been excluded from this law after a critic of the Bill had warned the government that dissecting readily became a 'mania' with medical men, and that to include them would undermine public confidence in hospitals.[62] Arguments had been raised in the South Australian parliament against including the destitute asylum, on the grounds that its inmates were mostly old and infirm, with few friends to look after them or consult their wishes, but no one mounted such a plea for those residing in lunatic asylums.[63] Critics did attempt to insist that positive consent to dissection must first be obtained, but the Attorney General responded that it would be 'inconvenient' to have to hunt up a wife or husband to seek their consent before a body was so used.[64] Under this statute, with hospitals excluded as a source of supply, it was South Australia's asylums that henceforth must provide most of the bodies for the University of Adelaide's medical school. After all, one journalist argued, those who lived in such places were of no interest or value to anyone outside the institution's walls.[65]

After 1884, it would prove to be particularly difficult for family members to claim relatives from asylums for burial. John Walton has argued that inmates of antipodean lunatic asylums were more likely than the general population to be isolated from kin, due to migration.[66] In this context patients could easily have 'no known relatives' recorded on their case file for, although it was in the interests of asylum officials to record family members to extract from them whatever fees they could contribute to a lunatic's upkeep and treatment, migration made this difficult. Thus, when a Justice of the Peace in the town of South Australian town of Oodnadatta committed one Mateo Jezfier to Adelaide's Parkside Lunatic Asylum on 15 July 1902, its medical superintendent Dr William Lennox Cleland sought to determine whether the man had relatives and was advised by authorities in Oodnadatta that Jezfier was 'a total stranger in these parts', where no-one had understood a word that the man spoke. 'No known relatives', Cleland wrote in Jezfier's file.[67] And twice each year—well after anyone could claim a corpse under the Anatomy Act—the government published a list of 'persons who died in the Parkside Lunatic Asylum . . . whose relatives were unknown or lived beyond the limits of the State'.[68]

ANTIPODEAN SPECIMENS

Two medical men who were the keys to corpse procurement in Adelaide had learned their anatomy from Professor William Turner in Edinburgh, during the period in which Turner was working closely with anatomy inspector James Russell to open up lunatic asylums as sources of supply in Scotland. One was Dr William Lennox Cleland at Parkside. The other was Dr William Ramsay Smith, South Australia's anatomy inspector. Under Cleland's superintendence, by the end of the century Parkside Lunatic Asylum had become the single largest source of subjects for dissection in South

Australia. Between November 1899 (when the colony's Chief Secretary first authorised Cleland to dispose of asylum corpses in this way) and August 1903, Cleland authorised the disposal of 71 bodies from its mortuary to the University of Adelaide's medical school, where he also held the post of Lecturer in Insanity (1902–1911).[69] Though the Anatomy Act also authorised dissections to be performed in the asylum mortuary, Cleland had not applied for a licence to do that. This meant that any dissection—as opposed to a post-mortem examination—undertaken there would be unlawful.

The way in which bodies and specimens were gathered at Parkside was exposed in 1903 during a government enquiry held to examine Dr William Ramsay Smith's activities with the dead. He had been taking possession of corpses and body parts, and sent many 'across the seas' to Scotland. Some went to Professor William Turner's museum at the University of Edinburgh, while others were shipped to the museum of that city's Royal College of Surgeons. I have examined these activities in depth elsewhere, and here focus specifically on one form of collecting inside the Parkside asylum—parts taken from the bodies of patients of Chinese, Indian and Aboriginal descent.[70] This enquiry revealed that William Cleland assisted Smith to use that asylum's mortuary as a place in which he could obtain the specimens he most desired, for both pathological and anthropological collections.

Working under the Anatomy Act, Cleland disposed of the bodies of every patient who died in the Parkside Lunatic Asylum without friends to the University of Adelaide's medical school to be dissected. Thus, when a young girl died at Parkside Asylum soon after her skull had been trephined at the Adelaide Hospital, Smith—who was the city coroner in addition to being the anatomy inspector—held an inquest into her death. Then he personally autopsied the corpse, removing the girl's skull cap and brain to send to Dr Charles Cathcart at the Royal College of Surgeons of Edinburgh 'in the interests of science'.[71]

In addition, Smith's anthropological collecting became a focus of attention at the 1903 enquiry. It examined what had happened to the corpse of a long-term Parkside patient, Chun Ah Kiom. In November 1902 when this man died, William Cleland had turned his body into a subject for dissection by filling in the appropriate form and sending it to Smith in his role as anatomy inspector. But On receiving that form, Smith had telephoned Cleland to ask if he could 'dissect' the body himself, rather than authorise its removal to the medical school. Cleland agreed, and the following day Smith arrived at the asylum with a knife he had obtained from a colleague, telling the man he was off to 'bone a Chinaman'. This he did, in the presence of a group of interested spectators including William Cleland, who had never before witnessed such a procedure. Smith subsequently shipped Chun Ah Kiom's skeleton to Professor Turner in a box that also contained other anthropological specimens.[72]

Much was made at the 1903 enquiry of the 'scientific' nature of this work. Smith and Cleland boasted of having learned their anatomy in

Edinburgh, where museum conservators were always glad to receive 'rare and interesting' specimens. Cleland admitted that Turner asked his Australian-based former students to send him bones as gifts. Chinese bodies, Cleland explained, were difficult to find, as Chinese people attached 'very much importance to their dead'.[73] Smith's canny barrister, Sir Josiah Symon, led Cleland to assert that such specimen taking was a normal and desirable scientific activity rather than mere mutilation. Professor Turner was 'one of the most eminent men in the world in anthropology and pathology', his museum 'second to none in the world', and the University of Edinburgh medical school was a seat of anatomical and anthropological learning and collecting. Cleland agreed that men like Turner were 'glad to receive specimens, rare and interesting, from graduates and former students of the University', stating that he would not hesitate to send such donations himself knowing that Turner was 'specially desirous of making his collection thoroughly representative of the different races of men for purposes of bone study, and requests gifts of skulls and other bones from present and former pupils.'[74]

In making such requests, Turner was far from alone. British, European and American museums were accruing large anthropological collections that included specimens of Aboriginal Australian people, as part of a quest to understand differences between the races of humankind.[75] In 1862 the British Secretary of State had written to the Tasmanian Chief Secretary to alert him to the desire of the Directors of the Ethnological Museum at Oxford for two Tasmanian Aboriginal skulls, one male, the other female.[76] Two years later another request was received from London. William Flower—conservator of the Hunterian Museum—asked Tasmanian surgeon Dr William Lodewyk Crowther for 'a pair, male & female' of Aboriginal skeletons.[77] Provincial museums in Britain also sought such material.[78] And from Staffordshire, private skull collector Dr Joseph Barnard Davis wrote to a contact in Tasmania offering to instruct any hospital surgeon on how a skull could be cut from a corpse with nobody being the wiser, then sent to him.[79] Davis tirelessly sought such material through connections he forged with well-placed medical men in Britain's colonies, especially physicians and surgeons who held positions in hospitals and gaols. He wrote to the governor of the Cape Colony in the following terms. 'There are of course many methods of procuring [skulls] . . . but I think the surest is by requesting the aid of medical officers, who are spread abroad in the most suitable situations. The Dutch medical officers in their colonies seem never to let a skull escape their hands, where in hospitals, &c. it may be secured and prepared.'[80] In southern Africa, Davis also forged a relationship with Dr William Guyton Atherstone, medical officer of the gaol in Graham's Town, who promised to acquire skulls on his behalf. However, to Davis's fury, in 1859 he learned that the gaol's governor had ordered that no one was to interfere with prisoners' skulls. Davis reported the matter to Governor Grey, asking him to have the order rescinded. He informed Grey that,

> This is a far more stringent regulation than any which prevails in the public Institutions in this country. Indeed, were such regulations strictly observed there would be in a great measure, an end put to pathological science, the progress of medicine and surgery—as well as craniology. If the minds of the Natives be not sufficiently enlightened to allow of any use being made of the lifeless body, surely those of Europeans, settled in South Africa, should have overcome such prejudices.[81]

The argument that refusing medical men the opportunity to mutilate corpses during dissections and to collect specimens was irrational, unscientific, was also used to good effect at the 1903 Adelaide enquiry, where Cleland was questioned about his power at Parkside Lunatic Asylum to send asylum bodies to the University's medical school to be dissected. He stated that the only criteria he used to make that judgement was whether or not the patient's body was claimed. 'If the dead had no friends', Cleland informed the enquiry, the body would be sent to the medical school.[82] It became clear from his evidence that this was despite the fact that Cleland knew that particular patients would have abhorred that post-mortem activity on their corpses. Sir Josiah Symon suggested that it would be 'insufferable to a devout Hindoo' to be 'cut into little pieces for dissection', to which Cleland responded that had such a man had friends he would not have been sent to the school. 'It is simply the feelings of the relations that we study', he asserted, and that was the rule which operated in all hospitals in connection with anatomy.[83] There was nothing callous about it; the only 'mischief', Symon cheekily insisted, occurred when the practice became known—for then the feelings of the *public* were hurt.[84] The Board of Enquiry absolved Smith of any wrongdoing on grounds including that the Anatomy Act had not been contravened, as it only covered dissection and Smith's specimen collecting did not easily fit into a definition of that activity. In closing the case for the defence, Sir Josiah Symon argued that if any man had been 'guilty of acts worthy of a "Jack the Ripper" [he] should certainly be out of the Civil Service, and placed in Dr Cleland's care at the Parkside asylum,' but that his client William Ramsay Smith was not such a man.[85]

After this finding, Smith continued collecting specimens including to ship to Edinburgh, and Cleland now also took a more active role in this regard. For years, he had been annotating Aboriginal patients' files with descriptive anthropological information. When a man known as 'Jimmy' was admitted to Parkside in 1900, Cleland noted the transverse scars that extended across the man's abdomen and sternum, his 'coppery black' face, overhanging eyebrows, flat nose, retreating forehead.[86] After 1903 he further facilitated the collection of Aboriginal corpses from the Parkside asylum. As Fforde has shown, when Wanamuchoo died in the asylum on 27 October 1903 Cleland filled in the form required under the Anatomy Act to dispose of the body to the medical school to be dissected, doctoring it by writing that the skeleton was of 'great scientific value' and ought to be preserved for the Adelaide Museum rather than 'lost'. Somehow that skeleton subsequently came into William Ramsay Smith's possession and four years after the man's death Smith sent it to the University of Edinburgh's anatomy museum.[87]

By 1907 the anatomy museum at the University of Edinburgh also contained three preserved heads of Australian Aboriginal men, sent there by Smith and no doubt accommodated in the room known as Professor Turner's 'skullery'.[88] In that year, Professor Cunningham published an illustrated article on his examination of these heads, one of which had been obtained from the lunatic asylum in Adelaide. The death of 'Pokalbe, alias Boco' had been published in the *Advertiser* on July 21, 1905, when his name was amongst those listed as having died in the asylum in the year ended 30 June, 'whose relatives are unknown or reside beyond the limits of the state.' The label attached to this specimen gave it a more detailed provenance which Cunningham included in his article:

> Pokallie, alias Boco, was sent to the lunatic asylum on May 23rd, 1894, and died of organic disease of the brain on June 13th, 1905. On admission he was well nourished and appeared in good health. The two central incisors of the upper jaw were absent. He was in a state of melancholic stupor the whole of the eleven years he was in the asylum. He never spoke nor took the least interest in anything that went on around him, nor even resented the violence he sometimes received from a fellow-countryman.

Cunningham also recorded the University of Edinburgh's debt to its colonial collector William Ramsay Smith, who had made 'numerous valuable contributions' to the ethnological collection.[89]

In addition, bodies sent from Parkside Lunatic Asylum to the University of Adelaide's Professor of Anatomy, Archibald Watson, were harvested for parts to send to museums. In 1909 Watson shipped two Aboriginal bodies to Arthur Keith at the Hunterian Museum at London's Royal College of Surgeons. The first was that of 'Judy' or 'Ulimba'; the second was 'Loodnatti, alias Scotty'. Loodnatti's remains were accompanied by a piece of paper on which Cleland had written: 'Dear Professor Watson, The aboriginal sent to the School of Anatomy the end of August 1910 and called "Loodnatti alias Scotty" was received into the Asylum from Euro Bluff. He is said to have a brother at Yudnaperina.'[90] Cleland knew that Loodnatti had a relative. Nevertheless, he designated him unclaimed and sent his body to the medical school.

CONCLUSION

The unclaimed remains of people who died in lunatic asylums had an afterlife that served the interests of science in Britain and Australia. Without the consent of anyone other than asylum superintendents, they were furtively collected and removed to medical schools where students dissected them. These bodies were gathered under legislation that had made people who died inside institutions vulnerable to such a post-mortem disposal of their corpses. While initially in England and Scotland, workhouses and hospitals comprised the major sources of supply, lunatic asylums assumed an increasing role over the course of the nineteenth century; and when British-trained medical men subsequently practised in Australia, this is the culture of corpse procurement they brought with them. There, lunatic asylums were a source of supply from the earliest days of university-based medical education, under facilitating anatomy statutes, as no workhouses existed in these colonies to supply the schools.

At least on paper, dissections appeared to be distinctively different procedures to the post-mortem examinations that were also performed on asylum patients' bodies, in the interests of pathological anatomy. Notably, these autopsies were not regulated by statute law. However in practice the two procedures could not be neatly differentiated. Body parts were commonly cut from corpses and retained during both, also in the interests of science, for medical students learned their anatomy in museums as well as dissecting rooms. In addition, inside antipodean lunatic asylums other opportunities for collecting became possible. Museums around the world vied for anthropological body parts—to exhibit and for their research collections. They sought the kind of perfect specimens that could be obtained by medical men, who worked in the ideal conditions provided by dissecting rooms and institutions' mortuaries. This was a kind of collecting in which such men reigned supreme.

NOTES

1. Helen MacDonald, *Human Remains: Dissection and its Histories* (New Haven: Yale University Press, 2006), 13–27 (published in Australia as *Human Remains: Episodes in Human Dissection*, Carlton: Melbourne University Press, 2005).
2. Lisa Rosner, *The Anatomy Murders* (Philadelphia: University of Pennsylvania Press, 2009); Sarah Wise, *The Italian Boy: Murder and Grave-Robbery in 1830s London* (London: Jonathan Cape, 2004).
3. Ruth Richardson, *Death, Dissection and the Destitute* (Harmondsworth: Penguin, 1987).
4. *Hansard Parliamentary Debates*, 3d ser., vol. 9 (1832), col. 1152.
5. Helen MacDonald, *Possessing the Dead: The Artful Science of Anatomy* (Carlton: Melbourne University Press, 2010).
6. For a discussion of the Anatomy Act's neglect regarding body parts see Helen MacDonald, "Procuring Corpses: The English Anatomy Inspectorate, 1842 to 1858," *Medical History* 53 (2009): 388–389; MacDonald, *Possessing the Dead*, 105–106.
7. Jonathan Reinarz, "The Age of Museum Medicine: The Rise and Fall of the Medical Museum at Birmingham's School of Medicine," *Social History of*

Medicine 18, no. 3 (2005): 422. On the museum at Guy's Hospital's medical school, see MacDonald, *Possessing the Dead*, 102–109.

8. On the disposal of waste from medical schools' dissecting rooms, see Helen MacDonald, "A Body Buried is a Body Wasted: The Spoils of Human Dissection," in *The Body Divided: Human Beings and Human 'Materials' in the History of Medical Science*, ed. Sarah Ferber and Sally Wilde (Farnham: Ashgate, forthcoming).
9. For a full discussion of *R v Feist* see MacDonald, *Possessing the Dead*, 74–93.
10. Museum Archive Letters, 1915; Annual Report of London's Anatomical Committee, 1914, Royal College of Surgeons of England (hereafter RCSE).
11. John Burden to Medical Superintendent of the Lunatic Asylum Gloucester, 26 March 1867, Post Mortem Examinations—Law Officers Observations, MH 51/533 (hereafter MH 51/533), National Archives (Public Records Office; hereafter NA).
12. MacDonald, *Possessing the Dead*, 101.
13. Cursham to J. Wilkes, 4 January, 1864, MH 51/533, NA.
14. Anatomy Inspector to D. F. Tyerman Esq., 8 December 1857, Colney Hatch Lunatic Asylum, Anatomy Inspector's Outward Letter Book, Miscellaneous, 1842–1858, MH 74/15 (hereafter MH 74/15), NA.
15. Robert Boyd, "Tables of the Weights of the Human Body and Internal Organs in the Sane and Insane of Both Sexes at Various Ages, Arranged from 2614 Post-Mortem Examinations," *Philosophical Transactions of the Royal Society of London* 151 (1861): 241.
16. Alastair Compston, "On the Weight of the Brain and its Component Parts in the Insane. By J. Crichton-Browne, MD, FRSE, Lord Chancellor's Visitor," *Brain* 130, no. 3 (2007): 579–598. After leaving Wakefield, Crichton-Browne had co-founded the journal *Brain* in 1878. His two-part article appeared the following year: "On the Weight of the Brain and its Component Parts in the Insane," in *Brain* 1, no. 4 (1879): 504–518; and *Brain* 2, no. 1 (1879): 42–67. On the examination of such brains in Victoria, Australia, see Dolly MacKinnon, "Bodies of Evidence: Dissecting Madness in Nineteenth-Century Victoria, Australia," in Ferber and Wilde, *The Body Divided* (forthcoming). Porters often worked on the corpses of people who died in institutions—see MacDonald, *Possessing the Dead*, 211; and MacKinnon, "Bodies of Evidence."
17. Report Presented 3 July 1871, 1; Museum Reports 1863–1880, RCSE. On the origins of this museum, see Simon Chaplin, "Nature Dissected, or Dissection Naturalized? The Case of John Hunter's Museum," *Museum and Society* 6, no. 2 (2008): 135–151.
18. On such collecting in Australia, see Tom Griffiths, *Hunters and Collectors: The Antiquarian Imagination in Australia*, Studies in Australian History (Melbourne: Cambridge University Press, 1996).
19. Joseph Barnard Davis Papers, Notebook No. 6, September 1859 to 1 October 1860, MS 140:6, 60, Royal Anthropological Institute of Great Britain and Ireland.
20. Dr John Beddoe wrote in his memoir of taking Davis to the Bristol Infirmary in which Beddoe worked and showing him 'a Morlachian sailor from near Ragusa, whom I was trying to cure of gangrene of the lung, resulting from having been half-drowned—a fine, handsome fellow, but desperately ill. "Now," said my friend, "you know that man can't recover; do take care to secure his head for me when he dies, for I have no cranium from that neighbourhood." After all, the poor Morlach made a wonderful recovery,

and carried his head on his own shoulders back to the Herzegovina.' In MacDonald, *Human Remains*, 102.
21. George Cursham to Nairne, 1 January 1864; Cursham to J. Wilkes, 4 January 1864, MH 51/533, NA.
22. Spring Rice to Clement Jrasy, 7 January 1864, MH 51/533, NA.
23. Humphry to Spring Rice, 12 January 1864, MH 51/533, NA.
24. Resolution passed at meeting held 23 February 1877, attached to Clerk to the Visitors Office, St Nect, Hants, to Commissioners in Lunacy, 24 February 1877, MH 51/533, NA.
25. Office of the Commissioners in Lunacy to Fras G. Butler Esq., 26 February 1877, MH 51/533, NA.
26. Elizabeth T. Hurren, "A Pauper Dead-House: The Expansion of the Cambridge Anatomical Teaching School Under the Late-Victorian Poor Law, 1870–1914," *Medical History* 48, no. 1 (2004): 76. Hurren shows that of the 2,953 corpses dissected at Cambridge between 1870 and 1920, 231 were acquired from asylums (Fulborn Asylum 100, Colney Hatch Asylum 58, Three Counties Asylum 42 and the London County Asylum 31), 89.
27. Gifford to Byrne, 28 February 1899, 132, Letters and Papers Between Home Office and Anatomy Inspector, 1890–1904, MH 74/11 (hereafter MH 74/11), NA.
28. Pick to Home Office, 8 March 1899, MH 74/11, NA.
29. Ina Scherder, email message to author, August 26, 2010.
30. *Hansard Parliamentary Debates*, Commons, 3d ser., vol. 286 (25 March 1884), cols. 742–3.
31. The British Secretary of State had funded the building of funeratories, following the recommendation of the anatomy inspector and agitation by Edinburgh-based medical teachers. The association of teachers that agitated for the funeratories comprised both university and private anatomy school men, although the university representatives were less likely to attend association meetings than were the private school men. The buildings' maintenance was funded by local councils and the funeratory superintendent was in the employ of the association of anatomy teachers. For the funeratories, see MacDonald, *Possessing the Dead*, 31–33, 37–42.
32. "The Anatomy Act," (a petition to the House of Commons), *Provincial Medical and Surgical Journal* (1840–1842) 3, no. 5 (30 October 1841): 100.
33. Turner chaired the meeting that elected Russell to this twin role on 26 February 1881. Letter Book, Inspector of Anatomy for Scotland, MH 3/6 (1875–1882) (hereafter MH 3/6), 256, National Archives of Scotland (hereafter NAS).
34. "Address at the Opening of the Anatomical Department in the New Medical Buildings of the University of Edinburgh," 1880, 3–4, Special Collections, Nq.7.10, University of Edinburgh (hereafter UE).
35. R. J. Berry, "Chance and Circumstance," Unpublished Manuscript, 75, Medical Museum, University of Melbourne.
36. Cameron to Russell, 6 July 1881, 282–3, MH 3/6, NAS. For public views on human dissection, see MacDonald, "A Body Buried is a Body Wasted," forthcoming. Even medical men are on record abhorring the thought of specimens being collected from the corpses of people they loved. Surgeon George Guthrie wrote of the 'horror' a man would feel on learning that body parts taken from a relative were exposed in bottles 'for the contemplation of the learned and the gaze of the curious.' George Guthrie, *A Letter to the Right Hon. The Secretary of State for the Home Department, Containing Remarks on the Report of the Select Committee of the House of Commons on Anatomy,*

and Pointing Out the Means by Which the Science may be Cultivated with Advantage and Safety to the Public (W. Sams, London), 1829, 9.
37. Turner to Russell, 3 October 1885, 16. Letter Book, Inspector of Anatomy for Scotland (1885–89), MH3/8 (hereafter MH3/8), NAS.
38. Edward Brush, "Notes of a Visit to Some of the Asylums of Great Britain," *American Journal of Insanity* (January 1883): 278.
39. Rutherford to Russell, 11 October 1882, 46. Letter Book, Inspector of Anatomy for Scotland (1881–85), MH 3/7 (hereafter MH 3/7), NAS.
40. Cleland to Russell, 27 July 1888, 208. MH 3/8, NAS. Cleland had previously held the Chair of Anatomy and Physiology in Queen's College, Galway.
41. Rutherford to Russell, 22 April 1887, 127, MH 3/8, NAS.
42. n.d.1884, 118, MH 3/7, NAS. In London in 1909 a committee of teachers planned to send a deputation to the Local Government Board to argue that matters should be arranged in this Scottish way, through a London-based local government bill (Anatomy Correspondence re Supply: Deputation from Medical Societies 1909–1912, MH 74/39, NA, 'Alternative Scheme to be Presented by the Deputation to the Presidents of the Local Government Board', clipped to Memorial to the President of the Local Government Board, undated and unsigned).
43. Russell to Cleland, 8 February 1884, 176. MH 3/7, NAS.
44. Cleland to Russell, 27 July 1888, 208. MH 3/8, NAS.
45. Macleod to Russell, 16 April 1889, 284, MH 3/8, NAS. These Bills became the Edinburgh Municipal Police Amendment Act (1891) and the Glasgow Police Amendment Act (1890). They compelled such bodies to be placed 'at the disposal' of the anatomy inspector ('Memorandum on the Question of the Supply of Subjects for the Teaching of Anatomy and Operative Surgery in the Medical Schools of the University of London', presented to the Royal Commission on University Education in London, January 1912, Anatomy Correspondence re Supplies, 1913–1918, MH 74/41, NA).
46. Russell to Cleland, 9 August 1888, 209–210, MH 3/8, NAS.
47. Macleod to Russell, 16 April 1889, 284, MH 3/8, NAS.
48. "Anatomy Acts, Laws, Regulations etc," Copy of letter from Anatomy Department to Dr Campbell, 12 July, 1914, 377–462, UE.
49. Commissioners in Lunacy to Reverend Burden, 13 April 1867, MH 51/533, NA.
50. The schools—and their students—protested vociferously when they received autopsied bodies, arguing that these were too 'mutilated' to be dissected. See MacDonald, *Possessing the Dead*, 99.
51. George Robertson, "Hospital Ideals in the Cure of the Insane: A Statement of Certain Methods in Use at the Stirling District Asylum, Larbert," *Journal of Mental Science* 48 (1902): 263, 264.
52. General Board of Control for Scotland, Edinburgh to James R. Motion, Clerk to the Glasgow District Board of Control, 4 February 1915, 377–462, UE.
53. Copy of letter from Anatomy Department to Dr Campbell, 22 April 1915, 377–462, UE.
54. Robert Campbell to Professor Robinson, 23 April 1915, 377–462, UE.
55. Cited in Cressida Fforde, *Collecting the Dead: Archaeology and the Reburial Issue* (London: Duckworth, 2004), 73.
56. In chronological order, during the nineteenth century Anatomy Acts were created in Victoria (1862), Tasmania (1869), New South Wales (1881) and South Australia (1884).
57. In Victoria, no records remain to show the source of corpses at the University of Melbourne's medical school during its early decades, but by the late 1890s

the major source was the Melbourne Hospital. See Ross Jones, "Cadavers and the Social Dimension of Dissection," in *The Body Divided*, ed. Ferber and Wilde (forthcoming). The source of bodies during the opening year of the University of Sydney's medical school (1883) were hospitals and asylums. See MacDonald, *Possessing the Dead*, 167.

58. The Tasmanian statute was the exception; it allowed twenty-four hours. For this law and its peculiar circumstances see Helen MacDonald, "A Scandalous Act: Regulating Anatomy in a British Settler Colony," *Social History of Medicine* 20, no. 1 (2007): 39–56.
59. *Sydney Morning Herald*, March 12, 1881, 3.
60. The New Zealand law designated 'the surgeon of any hospital, the keeper of any lunatic asylum, and the keeper of any gaol' as persons in lawful possession of the bodies of those who died in these places (*An Act to Authorise the Establishment of Schools of Anatomy and for Regulating the Practice of Anatomy Thereat*, 1875). In 1884 this statute was amended to include in addition 'any officer of police' and 'keeper of any asylum or public establishment wherein destitute persons are housed' (*An Act to Amend "The Anatomy Act, 1875"*).
61. MacKinnon reveals that this amendment included instructions that a copy of the Act was to be posted in a conspicuous place in penal establishments and public institutions with the exception of lunatic asylums. See "Bodies of Evidence" (forthcoming).
62. Debates in the Houses of Legislature during the First Session of the Eleventh Parliament of South Australia, from June 5, 1884 to November 14, 1884, 16 September 1884, col. 987.
63. Debates in the Houses of Legislature, Legislative Council, 16 September 1884, col. 986. In contrast, elsewhere they did. In the same year in New Zealand, parliamentarian Mr Shrimsky argued with regard to reforming that country's anatomy statute that it was wrong to confine dissection (which benefited the human race) only to 'the bodies of unfortunate wretches, who had no families, and who might have died in lunatic asylums, gaols, or hospitals'. He considered it to be 'their misfortune that they should end their days in institutions of that kind', and sad that 'a final stroke should be given to them by giving their bodies up as a sort of exhibition' (*Hansard*, New Zealand Parliamentary Debates, House of Representatives, 26 September 1884, 47).
64. Charles Kingston, *Hansard*, House of Assembly, 7 October 1884, 1226.
65. *South Australian Register*, September 16, 1884.
66. Cited in Angela McCarthy, "Ethnicity, Migration and the Lunatic Asylum in Early Twentieth-Century Auckland, New Zealand," *Social History of Medicine* 21, no. 1 (2008): 49.
67. A. E. Williams to Cleland, 15 July 1902, Correspondence Files—Lunatic Asylums Office and Successors, 1897–1922, GRG 34/72, State Records of South Australia (hereafter SRSA).
68. For example, the *Advertiser* newspaper published such a list on March 1, 1901, of people who had died at the asylum during the half year ended December 31, 1900.
69. "Documents Authorising Anatomical Examination of Particular Bodies by the School of Anatomy with Related Papers," 26 August 1903, Colonial Secretary's Office, GRG 24/166, SRSA. The Faculty of Medicine had been established in 1885.
70. MacDonald, *Possessing the Dead*, 185–215.
71. Evidence Taken by the Board of Inquiry into Charges against Dr W. Ramsay Smith, 1903, GRG 24/67 (hereafter GRG 24/67), A46–7, SRSA. An 1862

scandal regarding the collection of specimens from patients' bodies at the Yarra Bend asylum in Victoria has been noted by Catharine Coleborne in "Exhibiting Madness: Material Culture and the Asylum," *Health and History* 3, no. 2 (2001): 105; it is also discussed in MacKinnon's forthcoming "Bodies of Evidence."

72. For Smith's activities on this body see MacDonald, *Possessing the Dead*, 198–202.
73. 8 September 1903, GRG 24/67, A39, SRSA.
74. Cleland to Symon, 8 September 1903, GRG 24/67, A38–9, SRSA.
75. See, for example, Moira G. Simpson, *Making Representations: Museums in the Post-Colonial Era* (London: Routledge, 1996), 173–189.
76. Chief Secretary's Department to Superintendent of Oyster Cove, 22 March 1862, CSD 44/18/175, Archives Office of Tasmania.
77. MacDonald, *Human Remains*, 114.
78. For example, the Manchester Museum (see Samuel Alberti, "Culture and Nature: The Place of Anthropology in the Manchester Museum," *Journal of Museum Ethnography* 18 (2006): 7–21.
79. MacDonald, *Human Remains*, 109.
80. Davis to Grey, 6 June 1858, Grey Letters Collection (hereafter GL), Auckland City Libraries (hereafter ACL).
81. Davis to Grey, 1 January 1859, GL, ACL.
82. Cleland to Parsons, 8 September 1903, A34, GRG 24/67, SRSA.
83. Cleland to Symon, 8 September 1903, A41, GRG 24/67, SRSA.
84. Symon, A41, GRG 24/67, SRSA.
85. *Advertiser*, 15 September 1903.
86. 'Jimmy', said to be aged forty, was admitted to the asylum on June 13, 1900. Cleland's notes reveal that his committal may have been due to an altercation with his employer rather than because he was insane: 'Speaks English fairly well says that Mr Giles of Cavoire sent him rabbit catching and then refused him tucker, so refused to catch rabbits and drove rabbits away. Denies drinking "fire water". Talks rationally apparently and gives fairly intelligible account of himself. Not emotional at present. Complains of no hallucinations. Quiet now' (January to August 1900, GRG 34/39/1, SRSA).
87. Fforde, *Collecting the Dead*, 50–51.
88. MacDonald, *Possessing the Dead*, 205.
89. D. J. Cunningham, "The Head of an Aboriginal Australian," *The Journal of the Royal Anthropological Institute of Great Britain and Ireland* 37 (January–June 1907): 47.
90. Watson to Keith, 10 November 1910, Museum Archive Letters 1910, RCSE.

10 The Anatomy Museum and Mental Illness

The Centrality of Informed Consent

D. Gareth Jones

INTRODUCTION

Anatomical interest in exhibiting psychiatric remains raises a number of challenging ethical issues. These centre on the extent to which 'informed consent' has, or has not, played a role in obtaining the bodies of the recently deceased for medical purposes. Such issues also focus attention on the degree to which the bodies and brains of the mentally ill have, or have not, been used to shed light on mental diseases and therefore mental illness. This chapter outlines and evaluates three models of practice in this field. In the first, the bodies of the mentally ill have been used without consent, but purportedly for useful ends. In the second, bodies have been obtained unethically without consent to allegedly achieve useful outcomes, including the alleviation of mental illness. In the third, the bodies of the mentally ill have been obtained with consent for specific research projects aimed at increasing our medical and social understanding of neurodegenerative conditions.

In this chapter, considerable attention is devoted to the use of unclaimed human bodies as prescribed under the law, since these have, historically, dominated the anatomical scene and continue to do so, to a lesser extent, today. By analysing different historical and contemporary practices, this chapter then highlights the need to reconcile the tensions between legally obtained bodies, issues of consent, and ethical practice. I show that the bodies of the mentally ill in New Zealand Asylums have been used indiscriminately, with no particular interest in researching the physiological aspects of mental illness *per se*. A disturbing modification of this approach emerged during the Nazi era in Germany when the bodies of those executed for political, religious and cultural reasons were used by anatomists for their own ends. The example most relevant to this book concerned the use of brains for neuroscientific investigations into various mental conditions. A far more judicious development is the study of bequeathed brains to brain banks with the specific intention of investigating brain disorders, such as Parkinson's disease and Huntington's disease. This theme is included because it serves to balance the contribution that anatomists are currently making to the elucidation of mental diseases in the human community.

Additionally, brain banks can be looked upon as the research museums of the present day.

IDENTIFYING SOME PROBLEMATIC ANATOMICAL ROOTS

The history of obtaining bodies for anatomical dissection is a hotly contested one. In the early nineteenth century in the UK the use of unclaimed bodies became the main conduit, as opposed to the earlier use of the bodies of criminals. Hence the Anatomy Act 1832 (UK) came into being, making poverty the sole criterion for dissection. Although no reference was made to hospitals or workhouses, it reflected widespread medical opinion that the use of the bodies of hospital patients with no relatives in a position to bury them would create little opposition. This indeed was the case, and workhouses continued as the major source of unclaimed bodies in the UK through to the early years of the twentieth century.[1] However, as this source of bodies began to dry up, an alternative prolific source of bodies emerged, namely, those of the mentally ill who had died in mental asylums. These were also unclaimed bodies, and they were to serve as the predominant means of obtaining bodies for dissection for much of the first half of the twentieth century. Only with the dawn of a new era—one marked by the role of bequests—were the mentally ill dying in mental hospitals buried with some respect and dignity.

It is interesting that the initial Anatomy Act 1875 (NZ) made provision for living persons to bequeath their bodies voluntarily, unless a surviving husband or wife, or known relative objected. In other words, bequests featured in New Zealand legislation throughout the latter part of the nineteenth century up to the time of the 1964 Act. Intervening amendments to the 1875 Act dealt with details regarding the persons who had lawful possession of the body. It was only with the 1964 Act that the voluntary donation of bodies emerged as the primary means of obtaining bodies. In spite of the theoretical possibility of bequests from 1875 onwards, the first definite record of a bequest was 1943, with others appearing sporadically throughout the remainder of the 1940s.[2] In view of these observations the new era referred to above was not legislatively driven, but emerged as a consequence of the confluence of a range of cultural factors, including the disappearance of a generation of colonial adventurers; changes in attitudes towards the mentally ill; the nature of mental institutions; and concerted efforts to publicise bequests by the widespread distribution of information leaflets to solicitors.

While the bodies of those from mental institutions were predominantly used for dissection, some of them were presumably used to prepare specimens for displays in anatomy museums. This cannot be proved, since the provenance of the body parts in anatomy museum displays was not recorded. However, they cannot have been obtained from any other source.

Consequently, there is little doubt that the vast majority of preserved specimens emanating from the first half of the twentieth century were derived from unclaimed bodies, with many of these originating from the bodies of the mentally ill. This theme places the anatomy museum squarely within the purview of this volume. It is the hidden face of the display of psychiatry in museums.

In her chapter in this volume, Helen MacDonald provides a number of pertinent case studies of what became of the remains of asylum patients' bodies in Scotland, England and South Australia. This builds on her insightful and disconcerting studies of the manner in which the remains of murderers, impoverished hospital patients, women and Aboriginal people were mistreated by surgeons and anatomists in the nineteenth and early twentieth centuries.[3] In doing this she has exposed the way in which anatomy inspectors both in England and Australia contravened the respective Anatomy Acts and encountered the debatable nature of what constitutes an 'anatomical examination'.[4] Deception lay at the base of these scandalous activities that were also shrouded in secrecy. The end result was a trafficking in the dead in a manner never envisaged by those responsible for the original formulation of the Anatomy Act 1832 (UK), and the other countries whose legislation was based on this act.

From the perspective of an anatomist, what is immediately evident historically is the lack of general interest in the source of bodies, even when treated far more circumspectly than those documented in the MacDonald studies. The use of the remains of the mentally ill has hardly been a topic of vital interest to anatomists, let alone to the general public. It may be that our current sensibilities have been sufficiently awakened that we now contemplate how this was allowed to happen on such an extensive scale. We need to be aware that this may well still be current practice in some countries, however, and that, if so, it continues to elicit little in the way of broad public interest or even concern. This chapter delves into why this may have been the case, and what it is about the ethos of anatomists that has allowed this to happen. This will necessitate painting on the broader canvas of the wide-scale use of unclaimed bodies, of which the mentally ill formed only a part, as opposed to the use of bequeathed bodies. This provides the context for understanding how it has been that the use of the bodies of the mentally ill has not been considered remarkable.

This chapter situates one aspect of the discussion in New Zealand, since its history of these practices provides a pertinent backdrop to the almost universally encountered attitudes of anatomists towards the use of unclaimed bodies. The views of these professionals in New Zealand up to the 1950s were not an aberration; indeed, anatomists adopted the use of bequests earlier than in many comparable societies. The attitudes themselves stem from the role given to informed consent: is it central or has it been relegated to a position of irrelevance? The international context is provided by two contrasting accounts: one from the Nazi era, with its blatant disregard of informed consent; and one from contemporary neuroscience research, with its use of brain banks that illustrate the potential for good when pride of place is given to informed consent.

A PARADIGM OF ANATOMICAL PRACTICE— THE 'CONTRIBUTION' OF THE MENTALLY ILL

There is detailed evidence tracing the source of bodies coming to the Anatomy Museum in the Otago Medical School in New Zealand between 1876 and 1960. This was the outcome of the Anatomy Act 1875 (NZ), with its stipulation that any party having lawful possession of the body of a deceased person could permit that body to undergo anatomical examination, on condition that the deceased had not objected to this during their lifetime, or a surviving spouse had not done so. Over this period the use of unclaimed bodies was central to the Anatomy Department's ability to undertake human dissection for medical education purposes. Between the years 1876 and 1886 all the bodies except two came from the Dunedin Public Hospital. It is interesting that the two exceptions came from the Dunedin Lunatic Asylum. The Benevolent Institution had fulfilled the role of the poor house and by 1900 had become the major source of corpses for dissection, but by the mid-1920s it had become of marginal importance, being replaced by a range of mental institutions.[5] The Medical Act of 1908 added the medical superintendent or other medical officer of a public institution to the Mental Health Act as a category of persons entitled to the possession of a body.

This modification of roles was due to the increasing influence of the Dunedin Lunatic Asylum, the forerunner of Seacliff Mental Hospital, which—with the exception of the two earlier bodies—first appeared as a significant source of bodies in 1897, although it was not heavily used until 1905. Between 1901 and 1920 Seacliff alone provided 141 of the 180 bodies received from a number of mental hospitals.[6] From 1916 to the late 1950s the supply coming from Seacliff was found to be inadequate and so was bolstered by bodies from at least five other mental institutions both locally and from throughout New Zealand. In this way, even as recently as the mid- to late 1950s the anatomy department was almost entirely reliant upon bodies sourced from mental hospitals and these, not surprisingly, were regarded by the anatomy department as a vitally important source of bodies. For instance, in 1940, twenty-two out of the twenty-four bodies received were from mental hospitals, as were all thirty-six bodies in 1942, and sixteen out of the seventeen bodies in 1948.[7] All this was to change in the late 1950s and 1960s when bequests replaced the use of unclaimed bodies. However, even this positive change should not blind us to the tenuous nature of the ethical base existing at the time.

The downturn in the supply of bodies in the decade between 1943 and 1952 elicited a steady correspondence between the Professor of Anatomy and the Directors General of Health and Mental Health, as well as the medical superintendents of both mental and public hospitals. The aim of this correspondence was to obtain as many unclaimed bodies as possible. This situation continued until the late 1950s, by which time it was realized that the supply could only be improved by increasing the number of voluntary bequests.[8] One gets the distinct impression that this move to bequests was more a pragmatic one than the outcome of careful ethical deliberation. What other avenues might have been explored had bequests failed to eventuate?

While we have no way of answering this specific question, it prompts us to reflect on the ethical significance of using unclaimed bodies in general, and the unclaimed bodies of the mentally ill in particular. Two successive superintendents of the Dunedin Lunatic Asylum described the inmates in such pejorative terms as 'the general mob', 'the insane poor', and 'incurable pauper lunatics'.[9] These were long-term patients who had nowhere else to go. These descriptions encapsulate the views of society (and the medical profession) in the first part of the twentieth century towards those who were poor and mentally ill, as they were perceived as lacking any significant value in life. In being both poor and mentally incapacitated they were doubly disadvantaged; their poverty probably lay outside their control, and their mental incapacity most definitely did.

The essential point about using unclaimed bodies lies in the lack of any informed consent prior to death on the part of the donors. In the case of the mentally ill, there is no way in which this could have been obtained, due to their mental limitations. Although unable to look after themselves during life and hence determine their future needs, after death they were entitled to, and deserved more, rather than less, care. Treating their remains as unclaimed, and denying them a dignified burial shortly after death, suggests that the converse was the case. On the other hand, the Anatomy Act 1875 (NZ) did not ignore the need for a decent burial. The body, both before and after anatomical examination, was to be transported in a decent coffin or shell, and when dissection had been completed was to be interred in consecrated ground or in an appropriate public burial ground within eight weeks of death. Nevertheless, even with these stipulations in place, the body was being used in ways that lay beyond the decision-making of the deceased or of those who could speak for the deceased, and in ways that most people would not have wished for their own bodies at the time of death. This use of patients' bodies points to a lack of moral concern on the part of those with responsibility for their welfare. Rather than being protected, patients were exploited by those who wanted their bodies for the purposes of anatomical study and teaching.

This trend demonstrates quite clearly that the anatomy profession at that time was not particularly interested in the mentally ill as such, and that there was a fundamental distinction between bodies used for educational purposes and those used for scientific study. One could argue that they were being exploited for a 'higher' cause, namely, the provision of human material for medical education. They were treated as 'a means to an end'. In the absence of the ready availability of an adequate supply of cadavers for dissection, there would have been no dissection, and hence no teaching of anatomy to medical students. That supply happened to be provided by the long-term mentally incapacitated in mental hospitals, without relatives available to claim their bodies after death. According to the Anatomy Act 1875 (NZ), there were twenty-four hours available to inform the anatomy inspector of the death, and the body could not be removed from the place of death for thirty-six hours. A death certificate was also mandatory. In practice, therefore, relatives had to claim the body within twenty-four hours. There is no stipulation about how relatives were to be informed of the death.

Traditionally, anatomists had been prepared to accept bodies from any legally legitimate source. Additionally, they had served as advisors in framing the legislation.[10] While there is no evidence to suggest that they set out to act in an unethical manner, pragmatism was the dominant driver. The lack of serious ethical analysis on the part of the anatomy profession opened the door to widespread use of the bodies of those who had languished in mental establishments, with no hope of cure or of ever being able to live in society.

As we look back today on this historical episode it is easy to be highly critical of what appears to have been the callous attitude of anatomists. It is pertinent, however, to ask what the options were at that time. While the psychiatric profession is now equipped with a veritable pharmacy of medications, from antidepressants to antipsychotics, from mood stabilizers to stimulants, plus anxiolytics and hypnotics, this was not the case when the mental asylums were at their forbidding height. Deinstitutionalisation of patients as a policy was not even contemplated at this time. Raising this query is not meant to presuppose a particular response, but if the use of unclaimed bodies had not been an option, the remains of the long-term institutionalised may have been treated in a more dignified fashion. But even here one has to bear in mind the sobering cases described by MacDonald, in which public hospital bodies were harvested for body parts during dissection.[11]

The background is that of the Anatomy Act 1832 in the UK, which was drawn up in response to the raft of deeply unsavoury elements within anatomy as its teaching contributions to medical education proliferated in the eighteenth and early nineteenth centuries in the British Isles and in Europe.[12] The details are well known: using the bodies of executed criminals, body snatching, and even murder. The world of the so-called resurrectionists and the plenitude of macabre stories surrounding the rapid transport of the recently buried from graveyard to anatomy dissecting room make for thrilling, if chilling, reading. By any standards the unethical nature of these escapades is scandalous.

The ground breaking Anatomy Act 1832 (UK), which formed the springboard for legislation elsewhere in the colonial world, reflected the widespread medical opinion that the least troublesome and most acceptable source of bodies for dissection, in the minds of the public and politicians, lay in the use of legally unclaimed bodies. The unclaimed bodies of the poor and the outcast from respectable society came to represent the paradigm of choice for many years to come, with very little attention being given to its ethical justification. The British compromise served as a model that was adopted by one country after another.

Therefore, why was the bequest route so readily bypassed? Some insight into the possible reasons for this are provided by an instance in Melbourne, Australia, in 1869, when the University of Melbourne Anatomy School sought to establish a source of corpses for dissection from a Benevolent Asylum. In response the inmates at the North Melbourne Benevolent Asylum protested against the proposed automatic use of their bodies for dissection after death. According to the *Argus* newspaper, 'the inmates felt that their last moments would be made more painful by their minds dwelling on the horrible and repulsive uses to which their remains might be subjected.'[13] In response, a later commentator retorted: 'I should rather think that the people who live on the bounty of the government ought to be pleased at being able to make some return to the public who have kept them for so long.'[14] This frequently encountered sentiment, voiced in various societies, applies both to the impoverished and to those with severe mental illness. The state has cared for them during life; and so their contribution to the state is to 'willingly' allow their bodies to be used for the advancement of educational purposes after death. The irony is that this could, in some circumstances, have been accomplished by discussion and informed consent. By failing to provide even the merest glimmer of such an opportunity, free choice was replaced by coercion.

This lack of ethical reflection has had a number of ongoing consequences. First, anatomists and allied health professionals came to rely excessively on the legality of a procedure at the expense of subjecting its ethical underpinnings to serious analysis. Consequently, in the absence of any such analysis, they failed to give thought to the most basic issues of consent, let alone informed consent in its more recent, sophisticated sense. As one compares the 1875 and 1964 Acts in New Zealand the most striking difference is the divergence in the emphases placed upon the use of unclaimed and bequeathed bodies. The two acts allow for both, and yet while bequests play a subsidiary role in the 1875 Act they occupy the primary position in the 1964 Act. For anatomists, with their dependence upon legal strictures, this change had immense ethical repercussions. Another contrast between the two acts lay in a subtle change to the wording. The stipulation against removing a body within 36 hours of death (1875 Act) was replaced by not commencing the examination within thirty-six hours of death (1964 Act).

The primary place occupied by legal, as opposed to ethical, drivers in the thinking of anatomists was to have ongoing consequences for many years to come. Anatomists were, and still are, ill-prepared for the varieties of ways in which bodies came to be unclaimed, extending well beyond the impoverished dying in hospitals. In a global context, many of these unclaimed bodies have come from mental institutions and government mortuaries, with the remainder comprising the bodies of those executed for political crimes and religious beliefs, and also of those dying in concentration camps.

The tragedy has been that the anatomy profession has not established any ethical strictures to prevent worse forms of exploitation from taking place. The performance of certain anatomists during the Nazi regime provides an extremely unsavoury illustration of what can happen when the legal use of unclaimed bodies does not occur within an ethical process. With this episode we begin to appreciate that the ethically dubious realms in which anatomists have moved since the eighteenth century led some of them into an apotheosis of evil as recent as seventy years ago.

AN UNETHICAL PARADIGM: THE NAZI PERIOD

The various pogroms in Germany and its occupied territories under the National Socialist regime from 1933 to 1945 resulted in an escalation in the number of people subjected to capital punishment.[15] The consequence for anatomy departments was that through their readiness to utilize the bodies of those sentenced to death and subsequently executed an abundance of bodies from a much wider variety of sources became available. Indeed, the German Ministry of Education issued a decree that from 1939 all bodies of the executed should be delivered to the closest Anatomical Institute for scientific use.[16] The result was that, besides bodies coming from legal proceedings in civilian and military courts, bodies were also supplied from concentration camps, prisons and psychiatric institutions.[17]

Departments of Anatomy in Germany took advantage of this potentially prolific supply of human bodies for both research and teaching, and current evidence strongly suggests that all of them used the bodies of the executed and also of other victims of the National Socialist regime.[18] The use of these bodies appears to have been independent of the anatomists' political views.

Some collaborators stand out. In Austria Eduard Pernkopf, Head of the Anatomy Department and Dean of the Medical School in Vienna, ensured that the Department received over 1,300 bodies of executed individuals.[19] Moreover, arrangements were made to coordinate the timing of the executions for when the Department required them. Once there, the bodies were used in dissection courses and also as a source of information for Pernkopf's anatomical *Atlas of Topographical and Applied Human Anatomy*.[20] This highly regarded atlas was first published in 1943, with second and third editions in 1980 and 1989 respectively, many years after Pernkopf's death in 1955. These later editions had different editors and the same translator from the German and were very favourably reviewed for the quality of the illustrations. In more recent years, however, continued use of the atlas has been hotly debated as the origin of the body parts on which the illustrations were based has been questioned and brought into the public arena. This epitomises very clearly the tension between anatomical excellence and ethical constraints—major constraints in this particular instance.

In Poland Hermann Voss, Dean of the University of Poznan, is known to have been enthusiastic about the number of executions in Poznan, since they provided sufficient bodies for his Institute as well as for similar institutions in Breslau and Konigsburg. Not only this, he was ecstatic at the beautiful results possible of the dissections on account of the freshness of the cadavers.[21] Besides using these bodies for dissection, Polish skeletons, Jewish skulls and plaster casts of Jewish heads were prepared and sold.

The actions of Professor Julius Hallervorden, a section leader at the Kaiser Wilhelm Institute for Brain Research in Berlin, highlights the complete lack of concern displayed by doctors about unethically obtained corpses for dissection when medical scientific advancement was their intention. He was a neuroscientist who collected the brains of the victims of the euthanasia program. His explanation is revealing in its explicitness: 'there was wonderful material among these brains, beautiful mental defectives, malformations and early infantile disease. I accepted these brains of course. Where they came from and how they came to me, was really none of my business.'[22] Hallervorden, himself, is reputed to have removed many of the brains collected from the extermination centre.[23] During 1942, he was able to dissect the brains of '500 feeble-minded individuals'. By March 1944, he had received 697 brains in all.

Hallervorden was committed to the study of these brains, and was driven by scientific and clinical curiosity. For instance, he refused the brains of schizophrenics and epileptic individuals—not out of moral indignation, but because he did not believe that they would provide any useful scientific information. He also expressed disappointment that he was provided with neither relevant medical notes, nor with the remainder of the corpses for postmortem examination.[24] As a result of his work, Hallervorden published 12 articles in scientific publications during the postwar years, and in seven of these he was the sole author.[25] The topics included cerebral palsy, microcephaly, various neural tumours, and the effects of carbon monoxide on the developing fetal brain. Deeply troubling as this work was, it is even more so to realise that after the war he was recognised for this and related work by his academic peers, and received an honorary doctorate in 1956, before retiring as an emeritus professor in 1966.[26]

The relevance of this instance for the present context is that some brains of the mentally ill were being studied for good ends. The aim was to elicit information that could, theoretically at least, assist in an understanding of a range of medical conditions, but also—more problematically—issues of dissection and race. Of course, the abhorrent way and circumstances in which these brains were obtained suggests that such an end is highly dubious. There is no way of isolating the evil practice from any good intentions—assuming of course that there were any good intentions.

The Hallervorden example highlights the ethical dilemmas implicit in the use of human material obtained from ethically questionable sources. This extreme example serves as a salutary reminder that the context within which human-based research is conducted is crucial. It is also noteworthy that there was a connection in some quarters between anatomy and the racial hygiene movement, so much so that some anatomists in their role as racial hygienists helped to facilitate sterilisation and mass murder.[27] While this was far from universal, it demonstrates the manner in which anatomy was open to being readily incorporated into a philosophical and political mentality that overrode all normal medical ethical demands. It demonstrates too that there is an intimate relationship between anatomy and the political system in which it exists, and that if anatomists are not prepared to question the dominant politico-ethical consensus they may end up indulging in profoundly inhumane practices.[28]

The overriding desire to work on 'high quality material', while justified in narrow scientific terms, may only be feasible by participating in tragically unethical practices. A balance has to be struck between scientific aspirations and clinical detachment on the one hand and empathy on the other, a balance that was so upset within the National Socialist medicine of Nazi Germany that its ultimate consequence was monstrosity.[29] In the twenty-first century China faces equally challenging issues governing ethically obtained bodies, and medical practice.

Neither should anatomists hide behind the claim that the practices in which they engage are legal; they were legal in Nazi Germany. What should have been queried was whether practices considered legal are ethical by any generally accepted notion of what constitutes ethical practice. In other words, anatomists have a responsibility to be both ethically aware and ethically astute, and not blindly accept the standards imposed by their political masters. Although the law may deliver up bodies for dissection, this does not mean that it is an ethical process. The immediate consequences for the practice of anatomy and even for the anatomists themselves may be negative; nevertheless, an ethical ethos is essential for the long-term health of the profession and its contribution to human welfare.

In reflecting on these tragic events, the underlying premise was the legitimacy of profiting from unclaimed bodies. While the use of such bodies does not lead inevitably to the ethical morass encountered in the anatomical practices undertaken in Nazi Germany, it may provide an environment which enables such activities. If anatomists had stipulated that they would limit their use of bodies to those bequeathed following free and fully informed consent, the practice of anatomy may well have come to a halt. Sadly, no such defense against horrendously unethical practices was to emerge.

CONTEMPORARY REFLECTIONS ON THE LEGACY OF UNCLAIMED BODIES

I have argued so far that the practice of using unclaimed bodies for anatomical purposes lends itself to exploitation. At the time of the major legislation governing anatomy departments and anatomical dissection in the first part of the nineteenth century, the option of using unclaimed bodies was a compromise that satisfied the medical profession and was able to obtain a political consensus.[30] It was not the only option available since bequests were known at the time and could have provided a workable system. Unfortunately, there was little ethical input into those debates, and unclaimed bodies became standard practice for the next 130 to 150 years even in countries where bequests are now standard. It is in the light of these outcomes that Richardson has argued that the Anatomy Act 1832 (UK) delayed the rise of whole body donation by a century, and was—in her words—'one of the most brutal and hated enactments ever to sully the statute book.'[31]

Unfortunately, this is not merely of historic interest, since the continuing acceptance of the unclaimed option has persistent implications within clinical as well as anatomical circles. Consider China and the use of the bodies of the executed. The poignancy of these dilemmas arises from the frequency of executions (approximately 3,400 per year) and the reasons for them, which include corruption, counter-revolutionary activities, and violent and non-violent crimes.[32] The use of organs for transplantation from executed prisoners is well known and has been acknowledged by the Chinese government, which has made attempts to restrict this practice especially for foreigners on tourist visas.[33] While it has been claimed that prisoners on death row volunteer their organs to society, the nature of the consent provided is highly questionable. The timing and manner of the execution—to facilitate the transplantation—also bring into question the integrity of the ethical system within which they are carried out. This practice is reminiscent of the efficient, synchronised, and streamlined process of the Nazis that established a timetable of execution that met the particular delivery demands of the dissecting room.

The use of the bodies of bodies executed prisoners for anatomical purposes is less well documented. However, in view of the ready availability of human material following executions it would be most surprising if some of these bodies did not find their way to anatomy departments for teaching and research. An unnerving pointer in this direction is provided by the plastination industry. While considerable consternation has been expressed at the twenty-first century plastinated specimens prepared by Gunther von Hagens for his Body Worlds exhibitions in Dalian, China, he assiduously asserts that the bulk of his preparations are from bequeathed bodies. The same cannot be said for the whole body plastinates prepared for Premier Exhibitions, organizers of Bodies: The Exhibition. These specimens, which tend to be young and have Asian features, are acknowledged by the organisers to be unclaimed. Premier Exhibitions has been investigated by the New York State Attorney General's office for failing to ensure that the bodies displayed were not those of Chinese prisoners who may have been tortured and executed.[34] Although Premier Exhibitions have assured the public that this is not the case, the lack of evidence led the attorney general's office to demand documentation stating the source of the body, cause of death, and the consent of the deceased prior to death before the bodies can be displayed in this manner. The need for appropriate informed consent was considered essential. In other words, the use of unclaimed bodies was queried, especially within the political context of contemporary China.

In surveying some of these contemporary incidents, there has been no reference to the mentally ill. This is simply because there appears to be no evidence of the extent to which they currently serve as a source of human material. Yet in view of the widespread continuing use of unclaimed bodies it would be surprising if they did not feature prominently, albeit unheralded, in some of the plastinated exhibitions. As with all other instances of the exhibition of the bodies of the mentally ill, they are not displayed because of anything they might contribute to an understanding of mental illness. Rather, they are exploited for other purposes altogether. This exemplifies the low regard in which they have been, and sometimes still are, regarded.

For the past 150 years or so, anatomists have prided themselves on abiding by the law, although MacDonald has uncovered some startling aberrations.[35] Unfortunately, anatomists have paid far too little attention to the ethical underpinnings of the legal requirements, let alone the ethical shortcomings, of some of the legal situations. The latter is all too clearly illustrated by the German experience in the first half of the 1940s, when the legal situation was based on unethical aspirations. For example, there was no requirement to seek the consent of the families of the executed for their relatives' bodies to be dissected, while it was forbidden to release the bodies of Jews, Poles and those executed for high treason to their relatives.[36] Less extreme, and yet in my estimation having potentially far more extensive repercussions, is current legislation in a number of countries mandating that the bodies of the unclaimed be removed to the local anatomy department. These include a number of American states (Maryland, Pennsylvania and Texas) and South Africa.

The dismissive attitude of anatomists towards the use of the unclaimed bodies of those at the margins of society has not been an aberration, but has represented the attitude of broader society. This use of bodies has been normalized within the profession, in the sense that, if one regards it as an evil, that evil has occupied the central ground within anatomy. While the use of unclaimed bodies may not in itself be sufficiently reprehensible as to be classed in this way, it has opened the door to reprehensible activities. This lies at the core of the normalisation process and it is a process that colours anatomy to this day.

When getting 'good' bodies for dissection becomes the overriding objective, the source of the bodies is inevitably seen as occupying a place of secondary importance alongside the drive to utilize bodies and body parts of the highest standard of preservation and fixation for teaching and research. One approach would be to draw up a continuum of relative moral acceptability in the utilization of bodies and body parts. In my view the continuum would extend from bequests at the most acceptable end to unclaimed bodies from alleged politico-religious criminals at the least acceptable end. Between these two ends the degree of relative acceptability may extend from use of the unclaimed bodies of the poor, through indigenous groups and the mentally ill, to non-political criminals towards the least acceptable end. The crucial question confronting the profession of anatomy is to determine where a line of demarcation to denote total unacceptability should be drawn. Currently, this is an unasked question, let alone an unanswered one.

BRAIN BANKS AS RESEARCH MUSEUMS

A contrasting picture is provided by the relatively recent rise of banks of human material, especially brain banks. These have elicited little interest among the general public, mainly because they seek little publicity outside a number of focused clinical and neuroscience communities. Brain banks are research resources, the repository of frozen fresh human brain tissue. They are only able to function with the active backing of community neurological associations, support groups, and the families of those suffering from the diseases under investigation. This is a far cry, then, from most of what has been discussed above, since all the tissue is freely given to the brain bank and the sphere of interest is firmly on the brain and neurological diseases. Only the brains are retained; the reminder of the body is left intact. In addition to brains from those with neurological or psychiatric conditions, brains from persons with no such conditions are also collected for comparison purposes, a critical aspect of any research program.

The number of brain banks is steadily increasing and they are now found in many countries. In some countries there are well-established networks to improve communication between them. The diseases that are the subject of research carried out using material from brain banks include Alzheimer's, Parkinson's, and Huntington's diseases, multiple sclerosis, epilepsy, motor neuron disease, stroke and schizophrenia. An early example of a research outcome was the discovery of deficient dopamine levels in the brains of patients with Parkinson's disease that led to the development of l-dopa treatment. Other breakthroughs have included the discovery and characterisation of the amyloid deposition in Alzheimer's disease, Lewy bodies in dementia, variant Creutzfeldt-Jakob Disease (vCJD) and the role of glutamate in schizophrenia.[37] Researchers are now using an array of tests such as imaging technology to pinpoint circuits in the brain that can then be studied using gene chips and related molecular techniques.

An allied but further development is the DNA Banking Network, such as that set up by the Medical Research Council in the UK (Porton Down and Manchester University). The aim in this instance is to identify genes that are risk factors for diseases. While it extends beyond mental diseases, this form of genetic epidemiology includes collecting samples from those with late onset Alzheimer's disease, multiple sclerosis, Parkinson's disease and unipolar depression.[38]

These are indeed the research museums of the future, museums that will have considerable repercussions for increasing the level of understanding of a range of distressing conditions, and that hopefully in turn will usher in a new era of enhanced therapeutic agents and approaches. Any future assessment of anatomy and related museums should classify banks of this description as functional research museums.

SOME ETHICAL CONSIDERATIONS

As one looks back on the instances described in this chapter, three distinct models have emerged. In the first (use of unclaimed bodies for educational purposes) the bodies of the mentally ill have been used without consent but for good ends. Nevertheless, those ends have thrown no light on an understanding of mental illness; that was not their intention. The mentally ill have been used after death as a means to an end, the end in this case being medical education. In the second model (the Hallervorden research), brains have been obtained by grossly unethical means in order to increase understanding of neurological and mental conditions. Theoretically, the ends have been good ones, although these have been severely compromised by the manner in which the brains were obtained. The third model (brain banks) utilizes brains obtained following informed consent with the goal of throwing light on the causes of neurodegenerative illnesses.

If one starts from the core ethical principles of justice, autonomy, beneficence and non-maleficence, it is clear that, with the exception of the third model—that of brain banks—the other two models have failed to uphold justice, autonomy and non-maleficence, on account of the manner in which the bodies or brains were collected. In both cases there may be an element of beneficence, in that the bodies or brains may be put to good uses, but this is very limited in scope. The ethical debate centres on the balance that can be achieved between the good emerging from anatomical study of unclaimed bodies or the bad when the scientific benefits of Hallervorden type of brain research are countered by the significant ethical loss implicit in the ways in which the bodies and brains were obtained.

My conclusion is that the losses outweigh the benefits in both instances. While the imbalance is far greater in the Hallervorden case than in the use of unclaimed bodies for educational ends, there is an imbalance in both situations. On the other hand, brain banks point to an ethical way of obtaining brains and subsequently conducting research on them. This is to be applauded and encouraged since the interests of those with severe neurological and psychiatric conditions are uppermost, both in the present and in the future. The brains of those who have died have been obtained in an ethical manner, paying due regard to their autonomy, and seeking to treat them in a just and fair manner. The goal is that of improving the health and quality of life of sufferers in the future, but in seeking to achieve this end, ensuring the welfare of sufferers in the present is uppermost.

The brain bank thus provides a model for the use of the bodies and brains of the deceased, based upon fully informed consent and driven by high clinical and scientific aspirations. A remaining challenge for those in charge of anatomy museums is to decide how best to deal with body parts obtained within quite a different ethical context.

The mentally ill have been shamefully exploited on far too many occasions in the past, and this is still possible in some current circumstances. It behoves those in charge of anatomy museums and similar institutions to rectify these wrongs by utilising the ever-increasing technologies at their disposal to improve the welfare of the neurologically and mentally impaired by ethical means.

NOTES

1. Ruth Richardson, *Death, Dissection and the Destitute*, 2nd ed. (London: Phoenix, 2001), 271.
2. D. G. Jones and S. Fennell, "Bequests, Cadavers and Dissections: Sketches From New Zealand History," *New Zealand Medical Journal* 104 (1991): 210–212.
3. Helen MacDonald, *Human Remains: Episodes in Human Dissection* (Carleton: Melbourne University Press, 2005); "A Scandalous Act: Regulating Anatomy in a British Settler Colony," *Social History of Medicine* 20 (2007): 39–56.
4. Helen MacDonald, "The Anatomy Inspector and the Government Corpse," *History Australia* 6, no. 2 (2009): 40.1–40.17; "Procuring Corpses: The English Anatomy Inspectorate, 1842 to 1858," *Medical History* 53, no. 3 (July 1, 2009): 379–396.
5. Jones and Fennel, "Bequests, Cadavers and Dissections."
6. Ibid.
7. Ibid.
8. Ibid.
9. John H. Angus, *A History of the Otago Hospital Board and its Predecessors* (Dunedin: Otago Hospital Board, 1984), 47–50, 70, 260.
10. Jones and Fennel, "Bequests, Cadavers and Dissections."
11. MacDonald, *Human Remains*; "A Scandalous Act"; "The Anatomy Inspector"; "Procuring Corpses."
12. Richardson, *Death, Dissection and the Destitute*, xv.
13. *Argus* (August 13, 1869): 5, quoted in Ross L. Jones, *Humanity's Mirror: 150 Years of Anatomy in Melbourne* (South Yarra, Victoria: Haddington Press, 2007), 84.
14. *Speculum*, no. 11 (October, 1887): 47, quoted in Ross L. Jones, *Humanity's Mirror*, 89.
15. S. Hildebrandt, "Capital Punishment and Anatomy: History and Ethics of an Ongoing Association," *Clinical Anatomy* 21 (2008): 8.

16. K. Mühlberger, "Die Belieferung des Anatomischen Institutes der Universität Wien mit Studienleichen in der Zeit von 1938–1946, in Akademischer Senat der Universität Wien, ed., *Senatsprojekt der Universität Wien: Untersuchungen zur Anatomischen Wissenschaft in Wien 1938–1945*, 29–66.
17. Christopher Redies and others, "Origin of Corpses Received by the Anatomical Institute at the University of Jena During the Nazi Regime," *Anatomical Record Part B: The New Anatomist* 285B, no. 1 (2005): 6–10; Hildebrandt, "Capital Punishment and Anatomy," 8.
18. S. Hildebrandt, "Anatomy in the Third Reich: An Outline, Part 1. Nationalist Socialist Politics, Anatomical Institutions, and Anatomists," *Clinical Anatomy* 22, no. 8 (2009): 883–893; "Anatomy in the Third Reich: An Outline, Part 2. Bodies for Anatomy and Related Medical Disciplines," *Clinical Anatomy* 22, no. 8 (2009): 894–905; and "Anatomy in the Third Reich: An Outline, Part 3. The Science and Ethics of Anatomy in National Socialist Germany and Postwar Consequences," *Clinical Anatomy* 22, no. 8 (2009): 906–915.
19. Daniela C. Angetter (On Behalf of the Senate Project of the University of Vienna), "Anatomical Science at University of Vienna 1938–45," *Lancet* 355 no. 9213 (2000): 1454–1457.
20. D. J. Williams, "The History of Eduard Pernkopf's *Topographische Anatomie des Menschen*," *Journal of Biocommunication* 15, no. 2 (1988): 2–12; Sabine Hildebrandt, "How the Pernkopf Controversy Facilitated a Historical and Ethical Analysis of the Anatomical Sciences in Austria and Germany: A Recommendation for the Continued Use of the Pernkopf Atlas," *Clinical Anatomy* 19, no. 2 (2006): 91–100.
21. Götz Aly, "The Posen Diaries of the Anatomist Hermann Voss", in *Cleansing the Fatherland—Nazi Medicine and Racial Hygiene*, ed. Götz Aly, Peter Chroust and Christian Pross, trans. Belinda Cooper (Baltimore: Johns Hopkins University Press, 1994), 99–155.
22. Quoted in Christian Pross, "Nazi Doctors, German Medicine, and Historical Truth", in *The Nazi Doctors and the Nuremberg Code: Human Rights in Human Experimentation*, ed. George J. Annas and Michael A. Grodin (Oxford: Oxford University Press, 1992), 37.
23. "Contemporary Lessons From Nazi Medicine", *Institute of Medical Ethics Bulletin* 47 (1989): 13–20; "Bioethics Attacked in Germany", *Bulletin of Medical Ethics* 61 (1990): 19–23.
24. Michael I. Shevell and Jüergen Peiffer, "Julius Hallervorden's Wartime Activities: Implications for Science Under Dictatorship," *Pediatric Neurology* 25 (2001): 162–165.
25. J. Peiffer, "Assessing Neuropathological Research Carried Out on Victims of the 'Euthanasia' Programme,",*Medizinhistorisches Journal* 34 (1999): 339–356.
26. Shevell and Peiffer, "Julius Hallervorden's Wartime Activities."
27. Hildebrandt, "Anatomy in the Third Reich: An Outline, Part 2," 900, 903.
28. Hildebrandt, "Anatomy in the Third Reich: An Outline, Part 3."
29. Hildebrandt, "Anatomy in the Third Reich", Parts 1, 2 and 3.
30. Richardson, *Death, Dissection and the Destitute*, 100–130.
31. Ibid., 421.
32. Hongda Harry Wu, *Laogai—The Chinese Gulag* (Boulder: Westview Press, 1992), ix–x; H. H. Wu, "Using Organs From Executed Prisoners is Unethical," in *Biomedical Ethics: Opposing Viewpoints*, ed. Tamara L. Roleff (San Diego: Greenhaven Press, 1998), 103–107.
33. Mark Magnier and Alan Zarembo, "China Admits Using Organs From Executed Prisoners," *Los Angeles Times*, November 17, 2006.

34. Michael Wilson, "'Bodies' Exhibitors Admit Corpse Origins are Murky," *New York Times*, May 30, 2008, http://www.nytimes.com/2008/05/30/nyregion/30bodies.html (accessed June 3, 2008).
35. MacDonald, "The Anatomy Inspector" and "Procuring Corpses."
36. Thomas Waltenbacher, *Zentrale Hinrichtungsstätten. Der Vollzug der Todesstrafe in Deutschland von 1937–1945. Scharfrichter im Dritten Reich* (Berlin: Zwilling, 2008), 219. Hildebrandt, "Anatomy in the Third Reich: An Outline, Part 1," 886–887.
37. Medical Research Council, *Brain Banking—Science,* http://www.mrc.ac.uk/Ourresearch/Resourceservices/UKBrainBanksnetwork/Brainbanking/index.htm (accessed May 20, 2010).
38. Medical Research Council, *UK DNA Banking Network*, http://www.mrc.ac.uk/Ourresearch/Resourceservices/DNAbankingnetwork/index.htm (accessed May 20, 2010).

11 The Material and Visual Culture of Patients in a Contemporary Psychiatric Secure Unit

Fiona R. Parrott

Studies of psychiatric collecting have tended to focus on the material and visual traces of institutional environments of the past, rather than privileging the traces and presence of patients inside these institutions. This chapter provides a counterpart to existing material histories by presenting findings from a study of the significance of patients' material and visual culture in an existing psychiatric institution. It draws upon data from an ethnography conducted during 2003 in a medium secure psychiatric unit in southern Britain where I interviewed and spent informal time with male and female patients and staff on two single-sex wards.[1]

In this chapter I highlight patients' attempts to make sense of their detainment through their own material cultures. Patients display mixed feelings towards how their possessions and activities define their situation, in circumstances which patients perceive to be uncertain, artificial and otherwise largely beyond their control. I also consider the staff-led practices of recollection, salvage and exhibition of things from the asylum and latterly the mental hospital, which formerly existed on the same site. These activities help give those working at the institution a sense of past and at the same time, a sense of a progressive future. By contrast, some patients felt estranged from their own pasts and their present life in the secure unit, feelings which may be expressed though their relationships to things. Through this contrast among others, the chapter aims to stimulate reflection on the coherence and rationale of psychiatric histories and collections and the type of material and social presence implied by objects and images in exhibitions, from the perspective of what the patient culture can tell us in particular.

BACKGROUND AND METHODS

Medium secure units in Britain owe their inception to a series of reports commissioned during the 1970s, which recommended that regional hospital boards should provide more secure facilities for those psychiatric patients who required them.[2] By the 1980s, the building of numerous small-scale psychiatric units, usually accommodating between 30 and 100 patients, had begun in earnest. Defined by their custodial security measures, these units form part of a range of in-patient provision for mentally disordered offenders, located between open wards and high secure hospitals. Most patients admitted to medium secure units have been convicted of offences such as assault, homicide, arson and sexual offences, and diagnosed with serious mental illness, typically schizophrenia, bipolar disorder and depression. They may have transferred from prison or other psychiatric units as well as from the community.

The research site, which is still operating, is located within an urban catchment area in southern Britain. The ethnic composition of the in-patient population was 43 per cent European origin, 33 per cent Caribbean origin, 11 per cent African origin, 3 per cent South Asian origin and 10 per cent 'other', and patients' ages ranged from 18 to 45. Seventeen per cent of admissions were female while 83 per cent were male, which reflects the small number of women patients in forensic settings.[3] At the time of the study, the average length of stay was around two years.

A series of semi-structured interviews were conducted with all those who gave their consent on the women's ward and one men's ward (seven out of eight women from the women's ward, and twelve out of fifteen men). As part of these interviews I visited patients' rooms and talked about the things they kept in that space and the time spent there.[4] I spent time informally with all patients on the two wards at various times of day and early evening, attended hospital-wide events and interviewed nursing staff. The interviews were transcribed and analysed thematically alongside the contextual field notes.[5] The study was approved by the relevant medical ethics committees and all personal names have been changed to appropriate alternatives to protect patient and staff confidentiality. All participating patients were receiving treatment with anti-psychotic drugs.

INSTITUTIONS PAST AND PRESENT

In Britain, as elsewhere in the western world, most of the large mental hospitals and former asylums were closed down in response to the rise of community care. The secure unit visited as part of this study represents one of a number of regional forensic units designed for the detainment and treatment of psychiatric patients who have committed serious offences.[6] Patients are dependent on the medical profession in conjunction with the Home Office and mental health review tribunals to decree their length of treatment and detention. Their lives are bound up with the twin demands of confinement and medical care.[7] Traces of the past, however, persist amongst the built environment of the present, as this modern secure unit was built on the original site of an asylum established in 1895. The practices of 'history' around this site tell us something about its meanings in the later twentieth century.

At the beginning of the study, the brick water tower of the old mental hospital stood adjacent to the new secure unit buildings. During fieldwork this structure was demolished to make way for a housing estate. A ceremony was created to mark this event where current and former staff, members of the local community and a few patients gathered together to watch the tower collapse dramatically in a cloud of dust.

A succession of speeches and recollections were tied together by a narrative that emphasised improvements in care. One elderly woman who had worked as a nurse recalled patients' lack of privacy and personal space in the old mental hospital. The contemporary secure unit architecture and interior design are seen to realise an ethos of domesticity and caring that is directly opposed to images of institutions past, with their long corridors, strip lighting and open rows of beds. Bedrooms lead off short corridors, open plan sitting and dining rooms are furnished with sofas and television and soft lighting and paints in pastel blues, greens and yellows are thought to have a 'calming effect'.[8]

Positivist histories of progress have served to delineate these new styled units from their historical antecedents, recounting a transition from an age of restraint and fear to an enlightened realm of observation, diagnosis and therapeutics. Recognition of the needs and rights of patients or 'service users' was held up as an important area of advancement by the chief executive of the hospital, but is also a subject requiring future commitment. Finally, in order to preserve some of the present for future generations a 'time capsule' was buried next to a newly planted tree. This made explicit the intention to be remembered in the future.

As Catharine Coleborne's chapter in this volume shows, the phenomenon of psychiatric collecting and remembering the institution gained currency in the wake of deinstitutionalisation. Hospital closures prompted nursing staff in particular to collect what was, for them, the material culture of the workplace. The demolition of the last part of the former hospital and asylum established a similar salvage ethic. Among other things, staff found a large leather-bound hospital register from the end of the nineteenth century, containing black and white identifying portraits of patients, and entries describing each patient's mood, disposition and behaviour. This had been tossed into a builder's skip along with later photographs of the interior, including the sewing room and the recreation room. The service director, who saw them as a 'fantastic record that should never have been discarded,' arranged for a glass cabinet to be made and the objects displayed in the entrance hall of the psychiatric team base, commenting that

> there are terribly sad bits where people were incarcerated who would never have been today. You also get interesting snippets of the life of the people who provided care, for example, an incident where someone turned up drunk and was made to go home by the superintendent.[9]

The latest addition to the display cabinet was a gold and wood plaque awarded to the trust for service provider of the year. The incongruence of these objects highlights how the display of salvaged historic objects, alongside the contemporary award, is not simply about acknowledging the past as giving these psychiatric services a future. This reiterates the theme of the commemorative ceremony.

While staff and others see mementos and commemorative events as generating a sense of belonging based in and on the institution, granting them a glimpse into its historical antecedents and its (ideal) futures, patients are often engaged in using their relationships to things to dissociate themselves from what is present and orientate themselves towards other potential and contingent lives outside the institution. In the following sections I give examples of patients' attitudes and relationships to room decoration, clothing, photographs and mass media to show how these feelings are expressed, focusing in particular on the temporal and relational meanings of objects which affect their use by patients in this setting. These vignettes generate insights that complicate the ways in which 'psychiatric objects' are framed and discussed by patients themselves, and by hospital employees.

PATIENTS' MATERIAL CULTURES

Room Decoration

Some patients simply refused to decorate their rooms, saying 'it's not forever', as if fixing objects to the walls of these rooms metaphorically fixed them in the institution. In other words, patients tried to control the way they and their things became psychiatric objects and subjects. Attempts to try and help patients think of the unit as a home away from home included pictures hung high on the walls, televisions and recreational activities. These were complemented by more direct efforts to impress upon residents the need for them to accept being 'in here'. In contrast, most patients wished to assert that the institution was a temporary place to which they were unattached.[10]

The need to foster a sense of a transient space constrained normative practices of decoration employed in personal living areas.[11] The bareness of patients' bedroom walls could signify hope, but they also impressed upon patients the limitations of their situation. For some the walls of their room became the focus of conflicting desires. This ambivalence was illustrated by one patient's failed attempt at decorating. Christine, a British Jamaican woman in her forties, had been at the unit for three years and had no knowledge of when she would be able to leave. She described choosing some pictures from the computer and printing them with the intention of putting them on her wall. When she stuck them up she was faced with the evidence and emotional consequences of her work. She took them down, concluding 'It's not my home. My heart wasn't in it. I just want to leave here.'[12] This flimsy decoration, initially an expression of self-identity, came to imply that she had accepted the institutional room as her place, and was therefore deemed by her as not worth having.

Some patients justified certain decorations, by choosing some kinds of objects over others. This established a balance between comfort and an unwelcome sense of permanence. Ryan, a young British African man in his twenties, stated, 'Posters would be good but I don't wanna make it look like I'm here for a long time. I wanna make it look like, I dunno, it's my home for the meantime until I get a flat.' Purpose-made posters embodied an unacceptable level of intentionality so Ryan put up a few paintings of his own. 'They were only a quick thing. First I wasn't even sure I was gonna put them up on my wall. I just done them for something to do. Then when I looked at my room and my walls were bare, I just thought instead of keeping them for memory I would put them up.' He described putting these pictures up in a spontaneous, unplanned way. It may have been equally difficult to contemplate keeping them as mementos.

Items were indirectly used as a form of decoration by male and female patients, such as shoes lined up on a desktop or around the edge of the floor, or clothing hung off the front of a wardrobe. However, some patients regularly got rid of accumulated clothing—by having it removed to a relative's home—on the grounds that it was 'building up' and filling the space. Alternatively, little ways of taking over the space could be carried out, such as smoking a cigarette in the room or moving a piece of furniture. Activities such as moving a piece of furniture have been described as a non-presentational form of authorship over one's surroundings, but even this strategy was precluded by one man who retorted, 'leave it as it comes, it's not my home.'[13]

Talk of home and home decoration elicited strong emotional responses. Some of the strongest responses came from the women's ward. Although at first glance, some women kept many more things in their bedrooms than did their male counterparts, they measured these rooms against the labour and investment put into previous homes.[14] For Karen, a white British woman in her early thirties, 'home' was something that had been lost in the events which lead to her admission, which included an offence against her partner. When asked whether her room was homely she replied in monotone, 'It's not my home or my room, it's just somewhere to stay. Home's at home with my daughter and partner. I put a lot of work into my home, bought quite a lot of bits. It was my home—it won't be any more.'[15]

Carlton, a British Jamaican man in his forties, was among the few male patients who had settled in a council flat for seven years. When he first received unescorted leave he went to see his old flat, then occupied by another tenant. Carlton had lost every one of his possessions after he abandoned his flat—'when I got ill'—and the building itself was all that was left to see. Those patients who were close to discharge sometimes thought about their future home by planning and saving money to buy something for the future, 'to buy chairs and normal house furniture, so I can have my flat how I'd like it.' In short, patients asserted connections to past homes and to future homes, rather than furnishing their space in the institution. The problems with such memories and narratives, shaped through home-like objects, were the way these were characterised by disruption, discontinuity and loss. Imagined and actual futures were subject to uncertainty as much as hope.

Clothing

In contrast with patients' reticence towards decorating their rooms, some patients invested considerable effort in the expressive use of clothing within the institution. As noted above, patients felt freer to invest in clothing, even displaying it as a form of personalisation of their room. Clothes, shoes, jewellery and so on were things that were worn on a day to day basis. They were portable and transient, they moved with the person or were discarded, and, until they built up too much, they did not have the connotations of 'settling in' that proper furnishing and decoration had. As one patient joked, 'You can't go naked, can you!'

Huka, a woman of Somalian origin in her thirties, described how she would generate new looks: 'It's important to look after yourself. I change every day, my clothes, make up, you have to. Make it happiest for you. I do it for myself not anybody. I have a lot of jewellery, earrings, necklace. I change them all the time.' Some members of staff were surprised when Huka wore hats indoors or when she regularly dressed up to visit the cafe, 'like a teenage girl.' It was difficult for staff to perceive the way in which the institutional context framed these activities, as patients were not necessarily dressing in ways that were seen as suitable to the environment they were in.

Even other patients did not necessarily understand the rationale by which their fellow patients spent their money on clothing. Many patients received a means tested government clothing allowance of £150. On an escorted shopping trip, Carlton described how they went shopping for another British Jamaican patient, Courtney, who did not have leave, as well as himself. He was surprised by Courtney's choice, 'He give us a hundred and ten pound to buy one pair of trainers! It's them ones he's got on y'know. He's a bit doo-lally. Yeah well I told him with the money he spent on one he could a got at least three pairs. But he didn't seem to take much notice of me anyway. It's his money, he does what he wants with it.' It was not clear that other patients were the primary social context to which the expressive nature of dress was directed.[16] Karen confirmed this forcefully, saying, 'nothing really seems important, dress sense wise. I used to dress for other people. Being here on your own means I'm not really bothered.'

Several patients in particular were seen to eschew conventions of dress as the means by which bodies are made appropriate and acceptable within specific contexts.[17] Instead, the way they dressed seemed to have more relationship to their former home context and their external relationships. Another event involving Courtney illustrates the way unconventional behaviour may express those values. On one day during the height of summer, Courtney's brother had brought him a new fashionable coat. That the other patients sat in front of fans did not bother him; instead, he put on the coat, exaggerating his style of walking as he paraded around the ward. In this case clothing was used for self-expression and for interacting with peers in the unit, but these were consequences of Courtney's use of clothing and style which linked him to his brother and his home, including its music scene. Courtney showed me a photograph of himself and his sister in a local park close to their home, observing, 'See the clothes I'm wearing. They ain't changed a bit.'

Similarly, for the first year of her detention Huka was brought clothes 'all the time' by family and friends. I questioned whether the choices were always in her taste but she emphasised that 'they know what I like', demonstrating the established nature of her taste and style within these social networks. Where an expressive relationship to clothing was maintained, it was often because patients were able to direct this, not from their place in the institution, but through strong support by family and others outside the institution, in conjunction with shopping trips, catalogues, magazines and the media. In one woman's case it was church relationships and traditions that shaped her selection of clothing on Sundays both within the institution, and when she eventually had leave to visit the church. Such support, given form through clothing, gave these patients the resources to hold onto their identities in a world where they were uncertain.

The account of patients' relationship to clothing in this contemporary institution is quite different from Labrum's account of institutional clothing in this volume. This is not to say that patients' investment in clothing was always straightforward. Clothing also highlighted the extra weight which many patients gained during admission due to the combined effect of taking antipsychotic drugs, diet and taking limited exercise. As Huka admitted, 'the weight—I don't dress up like before . . . I've gone from a size 14 to 16, 18 to 20.'

Also in contrast to those who found themselves supported by their external relationships, Ryan liked 'nothing' about the clothes his mother and sister gave him, 'If it were me and I had community leave I could pick 'em myself.' In his case, his family could not make up for the curtailment of his own agency, as they chose things 'suitable' for his situation. He tried to resolve the issue by saying: 'you don't really need, you know, good clothes in here—it's better when you're out—when you've got more leave to the community is when you should have a lot of clothes—you know, you wanna look good in front of people.' Ryan implied that looking good in front of other patients, a disparate group of individuals on a single sex ward, was unnecessary. However, his mother's and sister's choices, and resources to buy him clothing, came to constrain Ryan's aspirations and imagination of another life beyond the institution. As he said, 'If I get one nice thing, I can use it as a goal or something.'[18]

Sometimes it can be the disposal of clothing that helps to stabilise identities, when these items of clothing are associated with unpleasant memories.[19] As introduced before, Karen had suffered considerable rupture in her roles as a mother and partner. She had spent several months on remand in prison. Her only agency with respect to her clothing had been to throw out every item she had worn in prison. In the psychiatric unit, her lack of effort in her dress became a marker of her separation from the outside world which Karen felt she had irrevocably lost at that time. A focus on clothing allowed some patients to establish continuities with life outside the institution on a day to day basis. However, the resources needed to engage in the construction of the self around clothing—with respect to an aspiration to be something beyond the institution—were not simply the clothes or accoutrements in and of themselves. Following on from this, we can see similar themes developed more directly through possessions such as photographs, cards and gifts.

Photographs, Cards and Gifts

Photographs, cards and gifts were important types of possessions because they depict the 'self-in-relation'.[20] Cherishing these possessions mediated relationships that were also sustained through visiting, phone calls and other forms of interpersonal contact. However, by virtue of being a material object they could also perform more autonomous roles: as memories of the deceased; as traces of former attachments; and as idealised companions or versions of those relationships.

Photographs, cards and gifts helped patients reconstruct themselves in the face of considerable rupture to their past social lives, bearing similarities with refugees' use of things to re-objectify themselves in a new environment.[21] The most common subject of photographs was people, including friends as well as families, though two patients also kept photographs of cars and homes. Gifts continue to presence the identity of the giver as an outcome of the exchange relationship,[22] and cards convey the relationship directly in writing and images.[23] As Sophie Chevalier has observed, keeping and displaying these items in domestic contexts allows an individual to signify collective belonging.[24] In this psychiatric secure unit, cherishing these things helped to repair the sense of social disconnection engendered by the secure institution and the gender segregated wards.

These personal possessions were an important resource. Carlton, the British Jamaican man in his late forties, was escorted to his mother's house every Sunday and therefore saw her regularly. He also saved every card his mother sent to him on each birthday and at Christmas. Carlton described how he would take the cards out of the black plastic bag which he kept hidden in his wardrobe and leaf through them as an antidote to the pressures of hospital life: 'They all locked away in my cupboard. But when I'm feeling down or whatever, I jus' pick them up and have a look at them.' These cards were an important source of support. Carlton felt valued by his mother who 'never once forgets to send a card' and used this experience to manage his emotions and counter his frustration with people in the unit. Rob, a young white British man similarly commented, 'I take the cards out from my drawer, you know, if I wanna remind myself that I got to do this, not just for myself.' While some displayed a photograph or card permanently, others kept their cards or photographs hidden in drawers, attesting to the private way in which they measured out these signs of affection or wished to contemplate these relationships. Any object could be a gift—from radios and televisions to soft toys, clothing and books—but their significance was hidden unless the association was narrated by the patient.[25]

Photographs also brought up complicated emotions as well as memories of the way family, partners and children were directly or indirectly affected by their illness, offence and detainment. Huka displayed photographs of a newborn baby, whose death prompted her detention, but she talked little about it. Some patients treasured a single photographic print that was all that connected them to their family. Sayeed, in his late teens and from a family of Somalian origin, showed me one such photograph of himself, his father and brother. He had carried it throughout his varied institutional experiences over the previous five years. The image had almost ceased to represent a moment in time, representing instead a constant ideal and tangible link to a family narrative. This narrative spoke as much to the potential of a life outside institutions as to its reality.

Some staff assumed that an intense attachment to things, as they saw it, evidenced their patients' impoverished ability to sustain relationships. By considering the specific objects and contexts of these attachments however, patients' emphasis on these important and tangible connections to both past and present relationships can be evaluated with regard to the people they connect to and, more generally, as relationships that expand their social world beyond the institution. These things are conduits to an alternative society to those of their peers and staff. The use of mass media, which I discuss in the final section of this chapter, was similarly put to use in mitigating the constraints of incarceration and loneliness.

Mass Media

Watching television and listening to the radio were prominent occupations among patients on the wards, noted by patients and researchers alike as a way of 'killing time' and combating boredom.[26] As Dolly MacKinnon emphasises in her chapter, it is important to understand the specific nature of recreational activities. Here, mass media was important as both a communal and a private activity. In communal space on the larger men's ward there was, invariably, at least one patient to be found in front of the widescreen television. From lunchtime onwards a group of men frequently watched the westerns shown in the afternoon. Communal acknowledgement extended to a flicker of shared amusement but, as often, shared boredom. The evening programming of familiar British and Australian soap operas, such as *Neighbours*, *East Enders* and *Coronation Street*, attracted a more convivial group which sometimes included members of staff.

Yet, as a communal activity, the ward television was subject to group decisions and rituals which could become problematic reminders of the imposed circumstances. Ian, a white British man in his thirties who had been transferred from prison, described watching the ward television, explaining that it meant 'having to say "do you want to watch this, do you want to watch that?" to other people.' When Ian sensed an argument brewing he would leave, 'so I say, well sod it. I'll go to me room and do what I want.' As Quirk and others have observed in their study of patients' strategies of risk management on acute psychiatric wards in London, in general TV rooms are less volatile places than some parts of the ward, but bedrooms offer a space for retreat.[27]

Watching or listening to media broadcasts in one's own room held specific attractions: it offered a form of companionship that was safe; one that was not directly connected to institutional life and allowed for the imagination of other lives; and one that was available day and night. Several patients described 'the chat' as the reason they tuned into the radio, and many listened to the radio or watched television in their rooms if they could not sleep. Carlton and Jane, a white English woman in her late thirties, described long term habits of lying in bed at night listening to specific radio shows. Carlton tuned to a Heart FM show that featured love songs and 'real life' love stories sent in by listeners: 'It's like if someone found a woman or a man, an' how they met them, an' they trying to get together. It's right interesting . . . 'Bout someone's love affair. They could 'a been in a club, or bibbed them in a car, met them, had sex with them, babies . . . ' Carlton considered the lives of those he heard about, recalling his own memories of relationships and thinking about his own desires. He asked himself, 'Would I do that?' and by comparison refined his own ideas about what makes 'a good relationship'. While these thoughts drew his attention to the limitations of detainment, this vicarious sociality experienced in memory and the imagination continued to constitute Carlton as a person with the capacity for sexual-love relationships. However, Carlton was quick to turn off shows, such as those broadcast on Friday evening, which emphasised getting ready to go out for the night.

On the women's ward, Jane described developing a more direct relationship to the two male presenters on her favourite show. She emphasised shared personality traits between herself and them, such as their sense of humour. Jane experienced the show as a conversation, a mode cultivated by presenters who speak to their listeners. In Jo Tacchi's study of domestic radio in Britain, she argued that from an experiential perspective, such imagined relationships impact upon one's sense of self and transform a person's reality, but she also noted that they were difficult to convert to different kinds of embodied interaction.[28] Jane regularly rang in and sent poems but she was severely disappointed by the presenters' lack of acknowledgement. Yet rather than stop listening, as Tacchi described, Jane framed her hurt in terms of a relationship: 'I'm pissed off with them at the moment.' Emphasising the importance of continuing the relationship, Jane overcame her periods of disappointment by devoting herself to more conventional interactions such as attempting to win competitions, which she did with significant success.

This use of radio is not specific to the secure unit but it was adapted to life in this setting. Radio shows, television soap operas, documentaries, up-to-date music shows and other types of broadcast could become the occasion for a release of certain kinds of desires, interaction and participation in a world of relationships that remained, relatively speaking, under their control and which continued to recall their capacity for deeper relationships of the kind they frequently perceived to be impossible or undesirable within the unit.[29] However, the notion of this engagement with media as a 'safe' form of sociability, lends itself to further consideration specific to ward life.[30] Dave, a white British man in his thirties, was a common target for bullying, particularly when other more dominating and aggressive men had run out of tobacco that week. Unsurprisingly, a routine of soap operas and narrative dramas watched on his tiny battery powered portable television occupied much of David's time inside his room. But this notion of safe sociability available in private rooms need not even be linked directly to the experience of bullying, as much as the dangers of expressed emotions on the ward.[31] Dave was not the only patient to note how they had to try to suppress anger or hurt in the unit, and in this case, soap opera could be an outlet for expressing emotionality, from sadness and anger to happiness.[32] As these examples show, fictional narratives and relationships to media personalities could help a patient 'get through' their time in the institution, through routines which existed within, but also beyond, the boundaries of the institution. This consideration of mass media adds to the previous discussion of decoration, clothing, photographs and cards, to show that throughout all their relationships to personal items, patients primarily tried to conceive of themselves in terms of another potential life—including actual and imagined relationships and spaces—outside the institution. They may be said to 'live within' these material cultures in complex and ambivalent ways. Therefore, these objects cannot be said to 'represent' institutional lives in any simple sense.

CONCLUSION

This chapter demonstrates how different ways of remembering, narrating and relating to material culture operate alongside each other in the lives of the staff and patients at a medium secure psychiatric unit in southern Britain. In particular, staff were interested in the traces of the past hospital and asylum which occupied the site. The last remaining piece of the old hospital architecture was demolished, providing an opportunity to remember the past and emphasise the important progress that had taken place. Some members of staff were keen to salvage portable pieces of this past, such as the patient register book and old photographs. They saw these artefacts as keys to their institution's former identity, with the interest in preservation and exhibition offering a means of reflecting on their own work identities. The nineteenth-century register offered a highly controlled and contained staff representation of patients in the institution, albeit one which is criticised by contemporary models of care, but it may do little to reflect the patients' perceptions of themselves within and beyond the asylum. Many of the staff have worked at the modern secure unit for a long time and invest considerably in their roles as part of a caring profession. Importantly, the work of recollection, presentation and display looks to the future as much as the past; in short, it helps give the institution both a past *and* future.

In contrast, many of the patients who were detained at the time of fieldwork were estranged from both their own pasts and their present life in the institution. Time inside doesn't count, in that it may not be valued. Instead, the ethnography demonstrated how patients frequently used their personal effects to construct links to an imagined or actual life outside of the institution. This may be accompanied by attempts to distance themselves from other resident patients. Patients have their own rooms and are allowed radios and televisions, other possessions such as photographs and clothing. They use these to forge connections to friends and family, to vicarious relationships to media personalities, and to engage with external trends such as changing fashions.

As we have seen, the problem is that these personal effects may not work as straightforward vehicles of identity. Rather, they are subject to extreme forms of ambivalence. While patients anticipate the future outside of the institution, they do not know how long they will be required to stay. The future is uncertain. Patients repeat the phrase 'it's not forever' in interviews. This is painfully materialised through some patients' reluctance to decorate their rooms. They may have wanted to display their own choices of decoration in their rooms, using furnishings, but feel strongly that this is not their home and such decoration or particular sorts of decorations should not be displayed. More transient goods, such as clothing, may make more appropriate means of maintaining links to home through style. The chapter has also showed how recreational activities such as watching television and listening to the radio were important means of filling time, countering silence and isolation by building alternative forms of society, including imagined romantic lives. Yet even these freedoms were likely to remind patients of the fact of their incarceration, such as radio programming on Friday nights which emphasised 'going out' into the mixed company of everyday life outside the institution.

If they look back to the past, many patients remember broken homes, lost access to children or the death of a child, and difficult memories surrounding the events and offence that led to their detention under the Mental Health Act (1983, amended in 2007).[33] Their possessions—for example, photographs of family members and children—may materialise these problems. Equally, possessions may become unintended mementos of their institutional stay. The politics of material presence and memory may be difficult to capture in psychiatric exhibitions, but this chapter provides a resource through which to think about these issues.

The focus on patients' material cultures demonstrated how patients' lives are lived within the tension between the desire to forget the past and deny the present; between hope and aspiration and lack of actual control over the future; and between the stability offered by the materialisation of personal identity and the oppressive nature of becoming too much 'at home' through the accumulation of goods inside. As this chapter has shown, some patients wished to leave as few traces of themselves as possible, choosing to personalise their space through activities such as smoking a cigarette. One wonders how these deliberately impermanent experiences should or could be explored through exhibitions of psychiatric objects and images used to evidence lives inside. As Alan Radley helps to clarify in his discussion of photographic representations of illness, the problem is not the need to take or exhibit more appropriate pictures or objects but to relate to the condition of the image construction as a representation, or the materialisation of experience, without unintentionally reducing the subject to the institution or illness.[34]

Through the contrast between my exploration of patients' material cultures and the institutional preservation of traces of psychiatric histories, this chapter provides a commentary on the coherence and rationale of psychiatric histories and the materiality of collections. First, this juxtaposition shows that, whereas collections are based on objects that are purposely collected and present, and which are seen to presence the institutional past, patients' lives and material cultures are governed far more by what is absent, transient and imagined. The implication is that when considering the relationship between psychiatric space, objects and memory of the past or present, this should be in the knowledge that the material and visual worlds of institutions are always mediations between multiple fragmented lives and locations. Second, history and narrative are as much about the future as the past. Here, patients' material cultures often resist coherence, while patients retain ambiguous and disjointed histories, memories and uncertain futures.

This is in contradistinction to the aims of staff or others who understandably may exhibit less inchoate artefactual and narrative histories of their institution's past and comparatively guaranteed future.

NOTES

1. Fiona R. Parrott, "'It's Not Forever': The Material Culture of Hope," *Journal of Material Culture* 10, no. 3 (2005): 248–249; "'Real Relationships': Sociable Interaction, Material Culture and Imprisonment in a Secure Psychiatric Unit," *Culture, Medicine and Psychiatry* 34 (2010): 559.
2. Home Office, Department of Health and Social Security, Butler Committee, *Report of the Committee on Mentally Abnormal Offenders* (London: HMSO, 1975), Command 6244.
3. Yonette Hassell and Annie Bartlett, "The Changing Climate for Women Patients in Medium Secure Psychiatric Units," *Psychiatric Bulletin* 25 (2001): 340–342.
4. Sarah Pink, *Home Truths: Gender, Domestic Objects and Everyday Life* (Oxford: Berg, 2004), 29.
5. Matthew B. Miles and A. Michael Huberman, "Reflections and Advice," in *The Qualitative Researcher's Companion,* ed. A. Michael Huberman and Matthew B. Miles (Thousand Oaks: Sage, 2002), 393–398.
6. Peter Snowden, "Regional Secure Units and Forensic Services in England and Wales," in *Principles and Practice of Forensic Psychiatry*, ed. Robert Bluglass and Paul Bowden (Edinburgh: Churchill Livingstone, 1990), 1375.
7. Tom Mason and Dave Mercer, "Rehabilitation: The Ship of Fools," in *Critical Perspectives in Forensic Care: Inside Out*, ed. Tom Mason and Dave Mercer (London: MacMillan, 1998), 131.
8. Abbey Hyde, "Secure Units: Caring Behind Locked Doors," *Health and Social Service Journal* 14 (1983): 440–442.
9. Personal communication (2010) from the Service Director of the medium secure psychiatric unit in Souther Britain, and research site for the study.
10. Parrott, "'It's Not Forever'," 250–251.
11. Judith Attfield, *Wild Things: The Material Culture of Everyday Life*, Materializing Culture (Oxford: Berg, 2000), 188.
12. Parrott, "'It's Not Forever'," 251.
13. Pauline Garvey, "Organized Disorder: Moving Furniture in Norwegian Homes," in *Home Possessions: Material Culture Behind Closed Doors*, ed. Daniel Miller (Oxford: Berg, 2001), 52–56, 65.
14. Ruth Madigan, Moira Munro, and Susan J. Smith, "Gender and the Meaning of the Home," *International Journal of Urban and Regional Research* 14, no. 4 (1990): 625–647.
15. Parrott, "'It's Not Forever'," 253.
16. Parrott, "'It's Not Forever'," 267.
17. Joanne Entwhistle, *The Fashioned Body: Fashion, Dress and Modern Social Theory* (Cambridge: Polity, 2000), 7–8.
18. Parrott, "'It's Not Forever',": 258–259.
19. Daniel Miller and Fiona R. Parrott, "Loss and Material Culture in South London," *Journal of the Royal Anthropological Institute* 15 (2009): 507–508.
20. Marianne Hirsch, *Family Frames: Photography, Narrative, and Postmemory* (Cambridge, MA: Harvard University Press, 1997), 2.
21. David Parkin, "Mementoes as Transitional Objects in Human Displacement," *Journal of Material Culture* 4, no. 3 (1999): 303–304.

22. Marcel Mauss, *The Gift: Forms and Functions of Exchange in Archaic Societies*, trans. Ian Cunnison (London: Cohen and West, 1954), 1–45.
23. Alexandra Jaffe, "Packaged Sentiments: The Social Meanings of Greeting Cards," *Journal of Material Culture* 4, no. 2 (1999): 115–141.
24. Sophie Chevalier, "Destins de Cadeaux," *Ethnologie Française* 28, no.4 (1998): 506–514.
25. Fiona R. Parrott, "Mais où a-t-on donc rangé ces souvenirs?" *Ethnologie Française* 37, no. 2 (2007): 307–308.
26. Dennis Gaffin, "From 'bugging-out' to 'chilling-out': Manipulating Emotion and Evoking Reason in a Forensic Psychiatric Hospital," *Culture, Medicine and Psychiatry* 20, no. 2 (1996): 217; Erving Goffman, *Asylums: Essays on the Social Situation of Mental Patients and Other Inmates* (London: Anchor, 1961), 45.
27. Alan Quirk, Paul Lelliott, and Clive Seale, "Risk Management by Patients on Psychiatric Wards in London: An Ethnographic Study," *Health, Risk and Society* 7, no. 1 (2005): 88.
28. Jo Taachi, "Radio Texture: Between Self and Others," in *Material Cultures: Why Some Things Matter*, ed. Daniel Miller (London: UCL Press, 1998), 25–46.
29. Parrott, "'Real Relationships'," 564.
30. Taachi, "Radio Texture," 25–46.
31. Gaffin, "From 'bugging-out' to 'chilling-out'," 199–228.
32. Parrott, "'Real Relationships'," 565.
33. UK Parliament, *Mental Health Act 2007 (Consequential Amendments), Order 2008*, http://www. legislation.gov.uk/ukpga/2007/12/contents/enacted.
34. Alan Radley, *Works of Illness: Narrative, Picturing and the Social Response to Serious Disease* (Ashby-de-la-Zouch: InkerMen Press, 2009), 15–42.

Contributors

Joanna Besley is Senior Curator at Museum of Brisbane. Some of the major social history exhibitions she has curated include Taking to the Streets: Two Decades that Changed Brisbane 1965–1985; Remembering Goodna: Stories from a Queensland Mental Hospital ; and Prejudice and Pride: Recognizing Lesbian, Gay, Bisexual and Transgender Lives in Brisbane. She writes articles and reviews in both academic and popular publications. Her most recent publication is (with Carol Low) "Hurting and Healing: Reflections on Representing Experiences of Mental Illness in Museums", in *Re-Presenting Disability: Activism and Agency in the Museum*, ed. Richard Sandell, Jocelyn Dodd, and Rosemarie Garland-Thomson, 130–142 (2010). In 2009, she was awarded a Churchill Fellowship to examine the role of museums in assisting communities to recover from traumatic events and experiences.

Barbara Brookes is Professor of History at the University of Otago. She is the author of *Abortion in England, 1900–1967* (1988) and editor of a number of edited collections. Most relevant to the asylum photography project is a book co-edited with Jane Thomson, *'Unfortunate Folk': Essays on Mental Health Treatment, 1863–1992* (2001). She has explored the on-going needs of the mentally ill in an article entitled "An Illness in the Family: Dr Maude Abbott and her Sister, Alice Abbott," in the *Canadian Bulletin of Medical History: Bulletin canadien d'histoire de la médecine* 28, no. 1 (2011).

Catharine Coleborne is an Associate Professor in History at the University of Waikato, Hamilton, New Zealand. She is the editor of several books including (with Dolly MacKinnon) *'Madness' in Australia: Histories, Heritage and the Asylum* (2003) and the author of several articles and chapters focused on psychiatry and museums. Her book *Madness in the Family: Insanity and Institutions in the Australasian Colonial World 1860s–1914* was published in 2010.

Mark Finnane is Professor of History at Griffith University, and currently ARC Australian Professorial Fellow and a Chief Investigator in the ARC Centre of Excellence in Policing and Security at the University. His doctoral research was on the history of mental hospitals and he has since published widely on the history of criminal justice, especially policing. His books include *Insanity and the Insane in Post-Famine Ireland* (1981/2003), *Police and Government: Histories of Policing in Australia* (1994), *Punishment in Australian Society* (1997), *When Police Unionise: the Politics of Law and Order in Australia* (2002) and *JV Barry: a Life* (2007).

Nathan Flis is completing his doctorate in Modern History at the University of Oxford, where his focus is the remarkably neglected career of Francis Barlow (c.1626–1704), England's first significant painter of birds and animals, and one of the country's most versatile artists before Hogarth. Nathan holds graduate degrees in history of medicine (McGill) and history of art (Oxford). His ongoing research interests include the visual culture of natural history, anatomy and psychiatry.

D. Gareth Jones is Director of the Bioethics Centre at the University of Otago, Dunedin, New Zealand, where he is also Professor of Anatomy and Structural Biology. Recent books include *Speaking for the Dead: The Human Body in Biology and Medicine* (2000/2009); *Designers of the Future* (2005); and *Bioethics* (2007). He is co-author with Alastair Campbell and Grant Gillett of *Medical Ethics* (4th edition, 2005). He is editor with Mary Byrne of *Stem Cell Research and Cloning* (2004), and with John Elford of *A Tangled Web: Medicine and Theology in Dialogue* (2009) and *A Glass Darkly: Medicine and Theology in Further Dialogue* (2010).

Bronwyn Labrum teaches in the School of Visual and Material Culture, Massey University, New Zealand. A former history curator at The Museum of New Zealand Te Papa Tongarewa, she first became interested in madness and asylums when completing her MA and produced foundational work in the field in New Zealand. She has since published widely on the related areas of women, mental health and welfare, including a chapter on welfare and society for *The New Oxford History of New Zealand* (2009). She has also published key works on museums, heritage and material culture, focusing on the collecting and display of clothing and other objects from everyday life over the twentieth century and the development of history as a museum discipline. Her abiding interest in clothing and fashion is apparent in her contributions to the Australia, New Zealand and the Pacific volume of *The Berg World Encyclopedia of Dress and Fashion* (2010).

Helen MacDonald is an ARC Future Fellow at the University of Melbourne. Her research focuses on the histories of human dissection, post-mortem examinations and organ transplants. Helen is the author of *Possessing the Dead: The Artful Science of Anatomy* (2010) and *Human Remains: Dissection and its Histories* (2006), which won the Victorian Premier's Literary Award (History category) and was short-listed for the Ernest

Scott History Prize. Her work is also published in journals, literary and science magazines. Helen is a member of the Advisory Boards of The Writing Centre for Scholars and Researchers and the Centre for Health and Society at the University of Melbourne.

Dolly MacKinnon is a Senior Lecturer in the School of History, Philosophy, Religion and Classics at The University of Queensland. She co-edited *'Madness' in Australia: Histories, Heritage and the Asylum* (2003) with Catharine Coleborne, and *Hearing Places* (2007) with Ros Bandt and Michelle Duffy. Her cultural history publications include "Music, Madness, and the Body: Symptom and Cure," *History of Psychiatry* 17, no.1 (2006); "'Amusements are provided': Asylum Entertainment and Recreation in Australia and New Zealand c.1860–c.1945," in *Permeable Walls: Historical Perspectives on Hospital and Asylum Visiting*, ed. Graham Mooney and Jonathan Reinarz (2009), and "'Bodies of Evidence': Dissecting Madness in Nineteenth-century Australia" in *The Body Divided: Human Beings and Human 'Materials' in the History of Medical Science*, ed. Sarah Ferber and Sally Wilde (forthcoming).

Fiona R. Parrott is a a NWO Research Fellow in Medical Anthropology at the University of Amsterdam. She has published her work with patients in a secure psychiatric hospital: "'It's not forever': The Material Culture of Hope" (2005), in the *Journal of Material Culture* vol 10, no 3, and "'Real Relationships': Sociable Interaction, Material Culture and Imprisonment in a Secure Psychiatric Unit" (2010), in *Culture, Medicine and Psychiatry* vol 34. She is the principal researcher on a study of 'Mental Health, Parenthood and Forensic Psychiatric Services in the UK'.

Nurin Veis has worked as the Senior Curator for Human Biology and Medicine at Museum Victoria for twelve years and is responsible for the curatorial content of the Mind and Body Gallery at Melbourne Museum. She has developed the exhibitions The Human Body and The Mind: Enter the Labyrinth, setting an international benchmark for exhibitions based on sensory and exploratory experiences. She has extensive experience in the ethical display of human remains as well as establishing guidelines for the ethical display of artworks by people who have experience of mental illness and trauma. She has a background in biochemistry, immunology and cell biology, having worked as a post-doctoral medical researcher in both Melbourne and New York.

David Wright holds the Hannah Chair in the History of Medicine at McMaster University in Hamilton, Canada. He has authored and co-edited eight books on the history of psychiatry, including, most recently, *Down Syndrome: The Biography* (2011). He is currently the principal investigator on a project researching the transnational migration of physicians in the second half of the twentieth century.

Bibliography

"Aboriginal remains repatriation." http://www.creativespirits.info/ aboriginalculture/people/aboriginal-remains.html (accessed November 18, 2010).

Alberti, Samuel. "Culture and Nature: The Place of Anthropology in the Manchester Museum." *Journal of Museum Ethnography* 18 (2006): 7–21.

Aly, Götz. "The Posen Diaries of the Anatomist Hermann Voss." In *Cleansing the Fatherland—Nazi Medicine and Racial Hygiene*, edited by Götz Aly, Peter Chroust and Christian Pross, 99–155. Translated by Belinda Cooper. Baltimore: Johns Hopkins University Press, 1994.

Angetter, Daniela C. (On Behalf of the Senate Project of the University of Vienna). "Anatomical Science at University of Vienna 1938–45." *Lancet* 355, no. 9213 (2000): 1454–1457.

Angus, John H. *A History of the Otago Hospital Board and its Predecessors.* Dunedin: Otago Hospital Board, 1984.

Antze, Paul and Michael Lambek, eds. *Tense Past: Cultural Essays in Trauma and Memory.* New York: Routledge, 1996.

Arnold, Ken. *Cabinets for the Curious: Looking Back at Early English Museums.* Perspectives on Collecting. Aldershot: Ashgate, 2006.

———. "Time Heals: Making History in Medical Museums." In Kavanagh,*Making Histories in Museums*, 15–29.

Atkinson, Katherine. "New Museum London exhibit pleads asylum: 'Cultivating Care' puts mental asylum stereotypes to rest." *The Gazette*, February 4, 2009. http://www.gazette.uwo.ca/article.cfm?section=Arts&article ID=2054 (accessed June 21, 2010).

Attali, Jacques. *Noise: The Political Economy of Music.* Translated by Brian Massumi. Manchester: Manchester University Press, 1985.

Attfield, Judith. *Wild Things: The Material Culture of Everyday Life.* Materializing Culture. Oxford: Berg, 2000.

Baird, George, researched by Robert Hill. "999 Queen: A Case Study of Government Demolition." In *The Second City Book: Studies of Urban and Suburban Canada*, edited by James Lorimer and Evelyn Ross, 70–95. Toronto: James Lorimer and Company, 1977.

Barthes, Roland. *Camera Lucida: Reflections on Photography.* Translated by Richard Howard. London: Flamingo, 1984.

BBC, Ouch! Disability Message Boards, Old Psychiatric Hospital Clothing. http://www.bbc.co.uk/dna/mbouch/F2322273?thread=3932070 (accessed January 16, 2009).

Belk, Russell W. *Collecting in a Consumer Society: Collecting Cultures.* London: Routledge, 1995.

Bennett, Tony, and Patrick Joyce, eds. *Material Powers: Cultural Studies, History and the Material Turn.* London: Routledge, 2010.

Berkhofer, Robert. *Fashioning History: Current Practices and Principles.* New York: Palgrave Macmillan, 2008.

Berry, R. J. "Chance and Circumstance." Unpublished Manuscript. University of Melbourne, Medical Museum.

Besley, Jo, and Carol Low. "Hurting and Healing: Reflections on Representing Mental Illness in Museums." In *Re-Presenting Disability: Activism and Agency in the Museum*, edited by Richard Sandell, Jocelyn Dodd, and Rosemarie Garland-Thomson, 130–142. London: Routledge, 2010.

"Bioethics Attacked in Germany." *Bulletin of Medical Ethics* 61 (1990): 19–23.

Blake, Eve. "Visiting the Asylum." *London Review of Books*, May 6, 2003.

Bloch, Maurice. "Internal and External Memory: Different Ways of Being in History." In Antze and Lambek , 215–233.

Boon, James A. "Why Museums Make Me Sad." In Karp and Lavine, 255–278.

Boon, Timothy. "Making the Modern World." *History Today* 51 (2001): 39–44.

Bourneville, D. M., and P. Regnard. *Iconographie Photographique de la Salpêtrière.* Paris: Progrès Médical/Delahaye, 1878. See http://jubil.upmc.fr/sdx/pl/toc.xsp?id=CH_00000124&fmt=upmc&idtoc=CH_00000124-pleadetoc&base=fa; see also http://openlibrary. org/b /OL20612739M/ICONOGRAPHIE_ PHOTOGRAPHIQUE_ DE_LA_SALPETRIERE.

Boyd, Robert. "Tables of the Weights of the Human Body and Internal Organs in the Sane and Insane of Both Sexes at Various Ages, Arranged from 2614 Post-Mortem Examinations." *Philosophical Transactions of the Royal Society of London* 151 (1861): 241–262.

Briggs, Asa. *Victorian Things.* Harmondsworth: Penguin, 1990.

Brookes, Barbara. "An Illness in the Family: Dr Maude Abbott and her Sister, Alice Abbott." *Canadian Bulletin of Medical History: Bulletin canadien d'histoire de la médecine* 28, no. 1 (2011).

Brookes, Barbara, and Jane Thomson, eds. *'Unfortunate Folk': Essays on Mental Health Treatment, 1863–1992.* Dunedin: Otago University Press, 2001.

Brunton, Warwick. "The Origins of Deinstitutionalisation in New Zealand". In "Histories of Psychiatry After Deinstitutionalisation: Australia and New Zealand. Special issue," edited by Dolly MacKinnon and Catharine Coleborne. *Health and History* 5, no. 2 (2003): 75–103.

Burke, Peter. "History as Social Memory." In *Memory: History, Culture and the Mind,* edited by Thomas Butler, 97–113. Wolfson College Lectures. Oxford: Blackwell, 1989.

———. *What is Cultural History?* Cambridge, UK: Polity, 2008.

Burns, Lawrence. "Gunther von Hagens' BODY WORLDS: Selling Beautiful Education." *The American Journal of Bioethics* 7, no. 4 (2007): 12–23.

Burns, Stanley B. *Patients & Promise: A Photographic History of Mental and Mood Disorders. Seeing Insanity: Selections from the Burns Archive, 1845–1945.* New York: Burns Archive Press, 2006.

Brush, Edward. "Notes of a Visit to Some of the Asylums of Great Britain." *American Journal of Insanity* (January 1883): 269–300.

Campbell, Alastair V., Grant Gillett and Gareth Jones. *Medical Ethics.* 3rd ed. New York: Oxford University Press, 2001. Campbell, Alastair, Grant Gillett, and Gareth Jones. *Medical Ethics.* 4th ed. Oxford: Oxford University Press, 2005: 49–71.

Cass, Daniel, and Lisa Cianci. *A Guide to the Records and Artefacts of the Kew Asylum Museum.* Melbourne: Australian Science Archives Project, 1996.

Chaplin, Simon. "Nature Dissected, or Dissection Naturalized? The Case of John Hunter's Museum." *Museum and Society* 6, no. 2 (2008): 135–151.

Charlton, James I. *Nothing About Us Without Us: Disability Oppression and Empowerment.* Berkeley: University of California Press, 1998.

Chevalier, Sophie. "Destins de Cadeaux." *Ethnologie française* 28, no. 4 (1998): 506–514.

Clendinnen, Inga. *Reading the Holocaust.* Cambridge University Press, Cambridge, 1999.

Clifford, James. *Routes: Travel and Translation in the Late Twentieth Century.* Cambridge, MA: Harvard University Press, 1997.

Clouston, Dr Thomas S., James Middlemass, and W. F. Robertson. "On the Typical Microscopic Lesions found in the Brain in Insanity: A Demonstration." *Journal of Mental Science* 40 (1894): 665–670.

Coleborne, Catharine. "Challenging Institutional Hegemony: Family Visitors to Hospitals for the Insane in Australia and New Zealand, 1880s–1910s." In Mooney and Reinarz, 267–308.

———. "Collecting 'Madness': Psychiatric Collections and the Museum in Victoria and Western Australia." In Coleborne and MacKinnon, *'Madness' in Australia*, 183–194.

———. "Exhibiting 'Madness': Material Culture and the Asylum." *Health & History* 3, no. 2 (2001): 104–117.

———. *Madness in the Family: Insanity and Institutions in the Australasian Colonial World, 1860–1914.* New York: Palgrave Macmillan, 2010.

———. *Reading 'Madness': Gender and Difference in the Colonial Asylum in Victoria, Australia, 1848–1880s.* Debut Book 2. Perth: Network Books, 2007.

———. "Remembering Psychiatry's Past: The Psychiatric Collection and its Display at Porirua Hospital Museum, New Zealand." *Journal of Material Culture* 8 (2003): 97–118.

———. "Space, Power and Gender in the Asylum in Victoria, 1850s–1870s." In Coleborne and MacKinnon, *'Madness' in Australia*, 49–60.

Coleborne, Catharine, and Dolly MacKinnon, eds. *'Madness' in Australia: Histories, Heritage and the Asylum.* UQP Australian Studies. St Lucia: University of Queensland Press, 2003.

Compston, Alastair. "On the Weight of the Brain and its Component Parts in the Insane. By J. Crichton-Browne, MD, FRSE, Lord Chancellor's Visitor." *Brain* 130, no. 3 (2007): 579–598.

"Contemporary Lessons from Nazi Medicine." *Institute of Medical Ethics Bulletin* 47 (1989): 13–20.

Corbin, Alain. *Village Bells: Sounds and Meaning in the 19th-Century French Countryside.* Translated by Martin Thom. New York: Columbia University Press, 1998.

Crane, Susan A., ed. *Museums and Memory.* Cultural Sitings. Stanford, California: Stanford University Press, 2000.

Crew, Spencer R., and James E. Sims. "Locating Authenticity: Fragments of a Dialogue." In Karp and Lavine, 159–175.

Crichton-Browne, J. "On the Weight of the Brain and its Component Parts in the Insane." *Brain* 1, no. 4 (1879): 504–518; *Brain* 2, no. 1 (1879): 42–67.

Cross, Simon. *Mediating Madness: Mental Distress and Cultural Representation.* New York: Palgrave Macmillan, 2010.

———. "Visualizing Madness: Mental Illness and Public Representation." *Television and New Media* 5, no. 3 (2004): 197–216.

Crowther, M. A. *The Workhouse System 1834–1929: The History of an English Institution.* London: Methuen, 1983.

Crowther, M. Anne, and Marguerite W. Dupree. *Medical Lives in the Age of Surgical Revolution.* Cambridge Studies in Population, Economy and Society in Past Time 43. Cambridge: Cambridge University Press, 2007.

Cunningham, D. J. "The Head of an Aboriginal Australian." *The Journal of the Royal Anthropological Institute of Great Britain and Ireland* 37 (January–June 1907): 47–57.

Dalley, Bronwyn, and Jock Phillips, eds. *Going Public: The Changing Face of New Zealand History.* Auckland: Auckland University Press, 2001.

Davies, Kerry. "'Silent and Censured Travellers'? Patients' Narratives and Patients' Voices: Perspectives on the History of Mental Illness since 1948." *Social History of Medicine* 14, no.2 (2001): 267–292.

Davison, Graeme. *The Use and Abuse of Australian History.* Sydney: Allen and Unwin, 2000.

de la Haye, Amy. "Introduction: Dress and Fashion in the Museum." In *The Berg Encyclopaedia of World Dress and Fashion, Volume 10: Global Perspectives,* edited by Joanne B. Eicher, 285–287. Oxford: Berg, 2010.

Dear, Michael J., and Jennifer R. Wolch. *Landscapes of Despair: From Deinstitutionalization to Homelessness.* Princeton: Princeton University Press, 1987.

Didi-Huberman, Georges. *Invention of Hysteria: Charcot and the Photographic Iconography of the Salpêtrière.* Translated by Alisa Hartz. Cambridge, MA: MIT Press, 2003.

Doessel, Darrel Phillip. "A Historical Perspective on Mental Health Services in Australia: 1883–84 to 2003–04." *Australian Economic History Review* 49, no. 2 (July 2009): 173–197.

Doessel, D. P., Ruth F. G. Williams, and H. Whiteford. "Deinstitutionalisation and Managerialism in Queensland's Public Psychiatric Institutions: Challenging 'Rhetoric' with Empirical Results." *Australian Journal of Public Administration* 68, no. 4 (December 2009): 459–483.

Dudding, Kathy, dir. *Asylum Pieces.* New Zealand, 2010.

Encyclopedia of Australian Science. "Charles Brothers Museum (1950s–1980s)." http://www.eoas.info/biogs/A002358b.htm (accessed June 22, 2010).

Entwhistle, Joanne. *The Fashioned Body: Fashion, Dress and Modern Social Theory.* Cambridge: Polity, 2000.

European Network for Indigenous Australian Rights (ENIAR). "Repatriation of aboriginal human remains." http://www.eniar.org/repatriation.html (accessed November 18, 2010).

Evans, Raymond. "Charitable Institutions of the Queensland Government to 1919." M.A. Thesis, University of Queensland, 1970.

Everett, Barbara. "Something is Happening: The Contemporary Consumer and Psychiatric Survivor Movement in Historical Context." *Journal of Mind and Behavior* 15, nos. 1 and 2 (1994): 55–70.

Fahy, Anne. "New Technologies for Museum Communication." In Hooper-Greenhill, 85–99.

Faulkhead, Shannon, and Jim Berg, with Lynette Russell, Ross L. Jones and Jason Eades. *Power and the Passion: Our Ancestors Return Home.* Melbourne, Victoria: Koorie Heritage Trust, 2010.

Ferber, Sarah, and Sally Wilde, eds. *The Body Divided: Human Beings and Human 'Materials' in the History of Medical Science.* History of Medicine in Context. Farnham: Ashgate (forthcoming).

Fforde, Cressida. *Collecting the Dead: Archaeology and the Reburial Issue.* London: Duckworth, 2004.

Finnane, Mark. *Insanity and the Insane in Post-Famine Ireland.* ACLS Humanities E-Book. London: Croom Helm, 1981

———. "Opening Up and Closing Down: Notes on the End of an Asylum." *Health and History* 11, no. 1 (2009): 9–24.

———. "The Ruly and the Unruly: The Uses of Isolation in the Management of the Insane." In *Isolation: Places and Practices of Exclusion*, edited by Alison

Bashford and Carolyn Strange, 89–103. Routledge Studies in Modern History. London: Routledge, 2003.

———. "Wolston Park Hospital 1865–2001: A Retrospect." *Queensland Review* 15, no. 2 (2008): 39–58.

Foucault, Michel. *Discipline and Punish: The Birth of the Prison*. Translated by Alan Sheridan. London: Penguin, 1991.

———. *Madness and Civilization: A History of Madness in the Age of Reason*. Translated by Richard Howard. New York: Routledge, 2001.

Fox, Daniel M., and Christopher Lawrence. *Photographing Medicine: Images and Power in Britain and America since 1840*. New York: Greenwood Press, 1988.

Frizot, Michel. "Body of Evidence: The Ethnophotography of Difference." In *A New History of Photography*, edited by Michel Frizot, 259–271. Cologne: Könemann, 1998.

Gaffin, Dennis. "From 'bugging-out' to 'chilling-out': Manipulating Emotion and Evoking Reason in a Forensic Psychiatric Hospital." *Culture, Medicine and Psychiatry* 20 (1996): 199–228.

Gardner, Jim. *Inside the Cuckoo's Nest: Madness in Australia*. Brisbane: Planet Publishing, 1977.

Garton, Stephen. *Medicine and Madness: A Social History of Insanity in New South Wales 1880–1940*. Kensington, NSW: University of New South Wales Press, 1988.

———. "Seeking Refuge: Why Asylum Facilities Might Still be Relevant for Mental Health Care Services Today." *Health and History* 11, no. 1 (2009): 25–45. http://www.historycooperative.org/journals/hah/ 11.1/garton.html accessed April 11, 2011.

Garvey, Pauline. "Organized Disorder: Moving Furniture in Norwegian Homes." In *Home Possessions: Material Culture Behind Closed Doors*, edited by Daniel Miller, 47–68. Oxford: Berg, 2001.

Gilman, Sander L., ed. *The Face of Madness: Hugh W. Diamond and the Origin of Psychiatric Photography*. New York: Brunner/Mazel, 1976.

Gilman, Sander L. *Seeing the Insane*. New York: Wiley, 1982.

Gittins, Diana. *Madness in its Place: Narratives of Severalls Hospital, 1913–1997*. London: Routledge, 1998.

Goffman, Erving. *Asylums: Essays on the Social Situation of Mental Patients and Other Inmates*. London: Anchor Books, 1961.

Griffiths, Tom. *Hunters and Collectors: The Antiquarian Imagination in Australia*. Studies in Australian History. Melbourne: Cambridge University Press, 1996.

Guthrie, George. *A Letter to the Right Hon. The Secretary of State for the Home Department, Containing Remarks on the Report of the Select Committee of the House of Commons on Anatomy, and Pointing Out the Means by Which the Science may be Cultivated with Advantage and Safety to the Public*. London: W. Sams, 1829.

Halbwachs, Maurice. *On Collective Memory*. Translated by Lewis A. Coser. The Heritage of Sociology. Chicago: University of Chicago Press, 1992.

Harvey, Karen. ed. *History and Material Culture: A Student's Guide to Approaching Sources*. Routledge Guides to Using Historical Sources. London: Routledge, 2009.

Hassell, Yonette, and Annie Bartlett. "The Changing Climate for Women Patients in Medium Secure Psychiatric Units." *Psychiatric Bulletin* 25 (2001): 340–342.

Health and Medicine Museums Special Interest Group (HMM). *Guide to Health and Medicine Collections, Museums and Archives in NSW and ACT*. Sydney: Special Interest Group, 2004.

Healy, Chris. *From the Ruins of Colonialism: History as Social Memory*. Melbourne: Cambridge University Press, 1997.

Healy, Michael. "Digital Public History: How Small History Museums Are Using the Web." Unpublished Directed Study, History Programme, University of Waikato, 2009.
———. "'No Easy Answer': Displaying Mental Health Histories in Local Museums." *Health and History* 9.1 (2007): 149–153.
Hides, Sean. "The Genealogy of Material Culture and Cultural Identity." In Pearce, *Experiencing Material Culture in the Western World*, 11–35.
Hildebrandt, Sabine. "Anatomy in the Third Reich: An Outline, Part 1. National Socialist Politics, Anatomical Institutions, and Anatomists." *Clinical Anatomy* 22, no. 8 (2009): 883–893.
———. "Anatomy in the Third Reich: An Outline, Part 2. Bodies for Anatomy and Related Medical Disciplines." *Clinical Anatomy* 22, no. 8 (2009): 894–905.
———. "Anatomy in the Third Reich: An Outline, Part 3. The Science and Ethics of Anatomy in National Socialist Germany and Postwar Consequences." *Clinical Anatomy* 22, no. 8 (2009): 906–915.
———. "Capital Punishment and Anatomy: History and Ethics of an Ongoing Association." *Clinical Anatomy* 21 (2008): 5–14.
———. "How the Pernkopf Controversy Facilitated a Historical and Ethical Analysis of the Anatomical Sciences in Austria and Germany: A Recommendation for the Continued Use of the Pernkopf Atlas." *Clinical Anatomy* 19, no. 2 (2006): 91–100.
Hill, Marguerite. "Madness in Early Twentieth-Century New Zealand: The Patient Case Records of Porirua Hospital, 1909–1915." Unpublished MA Thesis in Museum and Heritage Studies, Victoria University of Wellington, 2005.
Hirsch, Marianne. *Family Frames: Photography, Narrative, and Postmemory.* Cambridge, MA: Harvard University Press, 1997.
Hooper-Greenhill, Eilean, ed. *Museum, Media, Message.* Museum Meanings. London: Routledge, 1999.
Hunt, Suzanne "The Charles Brothers Mental Health Museum Collection Report," 1986. Museum of Victoria Research Library, Folder E, 1–2.
Hunter, R. M. "Historical Notes on the Auckland Psychiatric Hospital." *The New Zealand Nursing Journal* (February 1957).
Hunter, Richard, and Ida Macalpine. *Psychiatry for the Poor: 1851 Colney Hatch Asylum—Friern Hospital 1973: A Medical and Social History.* Folkestone: Dawsons, 1974.
Hurren, Elizabeth T. "A Pauper Dead-House: The Expansion of the Cambridge Anatomical Teaching School under the late-Victorian Poor Law, 1870–1914." *Medical History* 48, no. 1 (2004): 69–94.
Hutchinson, Mary, and Lea Collins. "Translation: Experiments in Dialogic Representation of Cultural Diversity in Three Museum Installations." *Museum and Society* 7, no. 2 (2009): 92–109.
Hyde, Abbey. "Secure Units: Caring Behind Locked Doors." *Health and Social Service Journal* 14 (1983): 440–442.
Jaffe, Alexandra. "Packaged Sentiments: The Social Meanings of Greeting Cards." *Journal of Material Culture* 4, no. 2 (1999): 115–141.
Johnson, Heidi. *Angels in the Architecture: A Photographic Elegy to an American Asylum.* Great Lakes Books. Detroit: Wayne State University Press, 2001.
Jones, D. Gareth. "Anatomical Investigations and Their Ethical Dilemmas." *Clinical Anatomy* 20, no. 3 (2007): 338–343.
———. *Speaking for the Dead: Cadavers in Biology and Medicine.* Aldershot: Ashgate, 2000.
Jones, D. G., and S. Fennell. "Bequests, Cadavers and Dissections: Sketches from New Zealand History." *New Zealand Medical Journal* 104, no. 912 (1991): 210–212.

Jones, D. G., R. Gear, and K. A. Galvin. "Stored Human Tissue: An Ethical Perspective on the Fate of Anonymous, Archival Material." *Journal of Medical Ethics* 29, no. 6 (2003): 343–347.

Jones, D. Gareth, and Maja I. Whitaker. *Speaking for the Dead: The Human Body in Biology and Medicine*. 2nd ed. Medical Law and Ethics. Farnham: Ashgate, 2009.

Jones, Karen, Eugen Koh, Nurin Veis, and Anthony White. With Rosalind Hurworth, Johanna Bell, Brad Shrimpton, and Anthony Fitzpatrick. *Framing Marginalised Art: Developing an Ethical Multidimensional Framework for Exhibiting the Creative Works by People Who Experienced Mental Illness and/or Psychological Trauma*. University of Melbourne: Custom Book Centre, 2010.

Jones, Ross. "Cadavers and the Social Dimension of Dissection." In Ferber and Wilde (forthcoming).

Jones, Ross L. *Humanity's Mirror: 150 Years of Anatomy in Melbourne*. South Yarra, Victoria: Haddington Press, 2007.

Joseph, Alun E., Robin A. Kearns, and Graham Moon. "Recycling Former Psychiatric Hospitals in New Zealand: Echoes of Deinstitutionalisation and Restructuring." *Health and Place* 15, no. 1 (2009): 79–87.

Kansas State Historical Society. "Straitjacket". http://www.kshs.org/ cool3/straitjacket.htm (accessed June 21, 2010).

Karp, Ivan, and Steven D. Lavine, eds. *Exhibiting Cultures: The Poetics and Politics of Museum Display*. Washington: Smithsonian Institution Press, 1990.

Kavanagh, Gaynor. *Dream Spaces: Memory and the Museum*. London: Leicester University Press, 2000.

———. "Remembering Ourselves in the Work of Museums: Trauma and the Place of the Personal in the Public." In *Museums, Society, Inequality*, edited by Richard Sandell, 110–122. Museum Meanings. London: Routledge, 2002.

Kavanagh, Gaynor, ed. *Making Histories in Museums*. Making Histories in Museums. London: Leicester University Press, 1996.

Kearns, Robin, Alun E. Joseph, and Graham Moon. "Memorialisation and Remembrance: On Strategic Forgetting and the Metamorphosis of Psychiatric Asylums into Sites for Tertiary Educational Provision." *Social and Cultural Geography* 11, no. 8 (2010): 731–749.

Kennedy, Marion. *The Wrong Side of the Door*. London and Wellington: George Harrap & Co., 1963.

King, Mary. *Truby King: The Man*. London: George Allen and Unwin, 1948.

Knell, Simon J., ed. *Museums in the Material World*. Leicester Readers in Museum Studies. London: Routledge, 2007.

Kordes, Doris. "The Arts of Care in an Asylum and a Community 1925–2004: Kenmore Hospital, New South Wales and Canberra, the Australian Capital Territory". Unpublished PhD Thesis, Australian National University, 2009.

Krupinski, J., A. McKenzie, and R. Banchera, eds. *Psychiatric Research in Victoria, Special Publication No. 9*. Melbourne: Mental Health Research Institute, Health Commission of Victoria, 1981.

Labrum, Bronwyn. "A Woman's World in a Male Universe: Treatment and Rehabilitation at the Auckland Lunatic Asylum, 1870–1910." In *New Countries and Old Medicine: Proceedings of An International Conference on the History of Medicine and Health*, edited by Linda Bryder and Derek A. Dow, 196–203. Auckland: Pyramid Press, 1995.

———. "The Boundaries of Femininity: Madness and Gender in New Zealand, 1870–1910". In *Women, Madness and the Law: A Feminist Reader*, edited by Wendy Chan, Dorothy E. Chunn and Robert Menzies. London: GlassHouse Press, 2005, 59–77.

———. "Dressing History Up: Introduction". In *Looking Flash: Clothing in Aotearoa/New Zealand*. Edited by Bronwyn Labrum, Fiona McKergow and Stephanie Gibson, 1–11. Auckland: Auckland University Press, 2007.
———. "The Female Past and Modernity: Displaying Women and Things in New Zealand Department Stores, Expositions and Museums, 1920s–1960s." In *Material Women 1750–1950: Consuming Desires and Collecting Practices*, edited by Maureen Daly Goggin and Beth Fowkes Tobin, 315–340. Farnham: Ashgate, 2009.
———. "Hand Me Downs and Respectability: Clothing and the Needy". In Labrum, McKergow and Gibson, 112–31.
———. "The Material Culture of Welfare in Aotearoa/New Zealand: A Case Study of Clothing". *History Australia* 2 (2005): 81.1–81.12.
———. "Material Histories in Australia and New Zealand: Interweaving Distinct Material and Social Domains." *History Compass* 8 (2010): 805–816.
———. "The Social Significance of Institutional Dress in New Zealand." In *The Berg Encyclopaedia of World Dress and Fashion, Volume 7: Australia, New Zealand, and the Pacific Islands*. Edited by Margaret Maynard, 332–337. Oxford: Berg, 2010.
Labrum, Bronwyn, and Conal McCarthy. "Museum Studies and Museums: Bringing Together Theory and Practice." *Te Ara Journal of Museums. Aotearoa: Special Issue: Museum Studies in New Zealand* 30, no. 2 (2005): 4–11.
Labrum, Bronwyn, Fiona McKergow and Stephanie Gibson, eds. *Looking Flash: Clothing in Aotearoa/New Zealand*. Auckland: Auckland University Press, 2007.
Lacan, Jacques. *The Four Fundamental Concepts of Psychoanalysis*. Edited by Jacques-Alain Miller. Translated by Alan Sheridan. The Seminar of Jacques Lacan 11. New York: Norton, 1988.
Le Goff, Jacques. *Histoire et Mémoire*. Paris: Gallimard, 1988.
Le Goff, Jacques, and Pierre Nora, eds. *Constructing the Past: Essays in Historical Methodology*. Cambridge: Cambridge University Press, 1985.
Leiberich, Peter, Thomas Loew, Karin Tritt, Claas Lahmann, and Marius Nickel. "Body Worlds Exhibition—Visitor Attitudes and Emotions.' *Annals of Anatomy* 188 (2006): 567–573.
Lewis, M. J. *Managing Madness: Psychiatry and Society in Australia 1788–1980*. Canberra: Australian Government Publishing Service, 1988.
Lipp, Martin R. *Medical Landmarks USA: A Travel Guide to Historic Sites, Architectural Gems, Remarkable Museums and Libraries, and Other Places of Health Related Interest*. New York: McGraw-Hill, 1991.
"Lives They Left Behind: Suitcases from a State Hospital Attic." The Willard Suitcase Exhibit Online. http://www.suitcaseexhibit.org/indexhasflash.html. (accessed March 2, 2011).
MacDonald, Helen. "A Body Buried is a Body Wasted: The Spoils of Human Dissection." In Ferber and Wilde (forthcoming).
———. "A Scandalous Act: Regulating Anatomy in a British Settler Colony, Tasmania 1869." *Social History of Medicine* 20, no. 1 (2007): 39–56.
———. "The Anatomy Inspector and the Government Corpse." *History Australia* 6, no. 2 (2009): 40.1–40.17.
———. *Human Remains: Dissection and its Histories*. New Haven: Yale University Press, 2006.
———. *Human Remains: Episodes in Human Dissection*. Carlton: Melbourne University Press, 2005.
———. *Possessing the Dead: The Artful Science of Anatomy*. Carlton: Melbourne University Press, 2010.

———. "Procuring Corpses: The English Anatomy Inspectorate, 1842 to 1858." *Medical History* 53 (2009): 379–396.

Macdonald, Sharon, ed. *The Politics of Display: Museums, Science, Culture.* Heritage: Care–Preservation–Management. London: Routledge, 1998.

MacKinnon, Dolly. "'A Captive Audience': Musical Concerts in Queensland Mental Institutions c.1870–c.1930." *Context* 19 (Spring 2000): 43–56.

———. "'Amusements are Provided': Asylum Entertainment and Recreation in Australia and New Zealand, c.1860–c.1945." In Mooney and Reinarz, 267–288.

———. "Bodies of Evidence: Dissecting Madness in Nineteenth-Century Victoria, Australia." In Ferber and Wilde (forthcoming).

———. "'Hearing Madness': The Soundscape of the Asylum." In Coleborne and MacKinnon, *'Madness' in Australia,* 73–82.

———. "'Jolly and fond of singing': The Gendered Nature of Musical Entertainment in Queensland Mental Institutions c1870–c1937." In Coleborne and MacKinnon, *'Madness' in Australia,* 157–168.

———. "Music, Madness and the Body: Symptom and Cure." *History of Psychiatry* 17, no. 1 (2006): 9–21.

———. "'Poor senseless Bess clothed in her rags and folly': Early Modern Women, Madness, and Song in Seventeenth-Century England." *Parergon* 18, no. 3 (2001): 119–151.

———. "'The Trustworthy Agency of the Eyes': Reading Images of Music and Madness in Historical Context." *Health & History* 5, no. 2 (2003): 123–146.

———. "The 20th-century mental hospital: A place in history but not in the adaptive reuse of surviving built heritage environments." Paper presented at "Green Fields, Brown Fields, New Fields," the 10th Australasian Urban History/Planning History Conference, University of Melbourne, February 7–10, 2010.

MacKinnon, Dolly, and Catharine Coleborne. "Introduction: Deinstitutionalisation in Australia and New Zealand." *Health and History* 5, no. 2 (2003): 1–16.

Madigan, Ruth, Moira Munro, and Susan J. Smith. "Gender and the Meaning of the Home." *International Journal of Urban and Regional Research* 14, no. 4 (1990): 625–647.

Magnier, Mark, and Alan Zarembo. "China Admits Using Organs from Executed Prisoners." *Los Angeles Times*, November 17, 2006.

Maroevi , Ivo. "The Museum Message: Between the Document and Information." In Hooper-Greenhill, 23–36.

Martin, Paul. *Popular Collecting and the Everyday Self: The Reinvention of Museums?* Leicester Museum Studies Series. London: Leicester University Press, 1999.

Mason, Tom, and Dave Mercer. "Rehabilitation: The Ship of Fools." In *Critical Perspectives in Forensic Care: Inside Out,* edited by Tom Mason & Dave Mercer, 129–145. London: MacMillan Press, 1998.

Mauss, Marcel. *The Gift: Forms and Functions of Exchange in Archaic Societies.* Translated by Ian Cunnison. London: Cohen and West, 1954.

McCarthy, Angela. "Ethnicity, Migration and the Lunatic Asylum in Early Twentieth-Century Auckland, New Zealand." *Social History of Medicine* 21, no. 1 (2008): 47–65.

Medical Research Council. *Brain Banking—Science.* http://www.mrc.ac.uk/ Ourresearch/Resourceservices/UKBrainBanksnetwork/Brainbanking/index.htm (accessed May 20, 2010).

———. *UK DNA Banking Network.* http://www.mrc.ac.uk/ Ourresearch/Resourceservices/DNAbankingnetwork/index.htm (accessed May 20, 2010).

Micale, Mark S., and Paul Lerner, eds. *Traumatic Pasts: History, Psychiatry, and Trauma in the Modern Age, 1870–1930.* Cambridge: Cambridge University Press, 2001.

Miles, Matthew B., and A. Michael Huberman. "Reflections and Advice." In *The Qualitative Researcher's Companion,* edited by A. Michael Huberman and Matthew B. Miles, 393–398. Thousand Oaks: Sage, 2002.

Miller, Daniel, and Fiona R. Parrott. "Loss and Material Culture in South London." *Journal of the Royal Anthropological Institute* 15, no. 3 (2009): 502–519.

Miron, Janet. "'In View of the Knowledge to be Acquired': Public Visits to New York's Asylums in the Nineteenth Century." In Mooney and Reinarz, 243–266.

———. "'Open to the Public': Touring Ontario Asylums in the Nineteenth Century." In Moran and Wright, 19–48.

Monk, Lee-Ann. *Attending Madness: At Work in the Australian Colonial Asylum.* Amsterdam: Rodopi, 2008.

Mooney, Graham, and Jonathan Reinarz, eds. *Permeable Walls: Historical Perspectives on Hospital and Asylum Visiting.* Wellcome Series in the History of Medicine/Clio Medica 86. Amsterdam: Rodopi, 2009.

Moran, James E., and David Wright, eds. *Mental Health and Canadian Society: Historical Perspectives.* Studies in the History of Medicine, Health and Society. Montreal and Kingston: McGill-Queen's University Press, 2006.

Mühlberger, K. "Die Belieferung des Anatomischen Institutes der Universität Wien mit Studienleichen in der Zeit von 1938–1946." In *Senatsprojekt der Universität Wien: Untersuchungen zur anatomischen Wissenschaft in Wien 1938–1945*, edited by Akademischer Senat der Universität Wien, 1998.

Museum of Brisbane. Filmed Interviews, *Remembering Goodna: Stories from a Queensland Mental Hospital* Exhibition. Brisbane, 2007–2008.

———. Visitors' Comments, *Remembering Goodna: Stories From a Queensland Mental Hospital* Exhibition. Brisbane, 2007–2008.

National Empowerment Center. Articles, "Peter Beresford on the need for a survivor-controlled museum of madness." 2008. http://www. power2u.org/articles/history-project/museum.html accessed April 1, 2011.

The Native American Graves Protection and Repatriation Act (NAGPRA), 1990. http://www.nps.gov/nagpra/ (accessed November 18, 2010).

New Zealand Centre for Photography. *http://www.nzcp.com/Features/tabid/122/* articleType/ArticleView/articleld/40/Historic-Cameras-Truby-King-and-Ed-Hillary.aspx accessed April 1, 2011.

Nichols, David, Dolly MacKinnon and Keir Reeves. "Goldfields Asylums: Anxieties, Evasions and Erasures." In *Deeper Leads: New Approaches to Victorian Goldfields History,* edited by Keir Reeves and David Nichols, 39–62. Ballarat, Victoria: Ballarat Heritage Services, 2007.

Nora, Pierre. "Between Memory and History: *Les Lieux de Mémoire.*" *Representations* 26 (1989): 7–24.

Nora, Pierre, ed. *Rethinking France: Les Lieux de Mémoire.* 2 vols. Translated by Mary Seidman Trouille and David P. Jordan. Chicago: Chicago University Press, 2001.

Nora, Pierre, and Lawrence D. Kritzman, eds. *Realms of Memory: Rethinking the French Past.* 3 vols. Translated by Arthur Goldhammer. New York: Columbia University Press, 1996–1998.

———. *Realms of Memory: Rethinking the French Past.* Vol. 3: Symbols. Translated by Arthur Goldhammer. New York: Columbia University Press, 1998.

O'Boyle, Shaun. "Modern Ruins–Portaits of Place." "Asylums." "'Byberry' & 'Buffalo'." http://oboylephoto.com/byberry/ index.htm; http://oboylephoto.com/buffalo/index.htm. (accessed March 1, 2011).

Olsen, Bjørnar. "Material Culture After Text: Re-Membering Things." *Norwegian Archaeological Review* 36, no. 2 (2003): 87–104.

Osborne, Ray. "Asylums as Cultural Heritage: The Challenges of Adaptive Re-Use." In Coleborne and MacKinnon, *'Madness' in Australia*, 217–229.

Paisley, Fiona. "Peeling Back History: The Remembering Goodna Exhibition." *Health and History* 11, no. 1 (2009): 172–179.

Parkin, David. "Mementoes as Transitional Objects in Human Displacement." *Journal of Material Culture* 4, no. 3 (1999): 303–320.

Parr, Hester. "Bodies and Psychiatric Medicine: Interpreting Different Geographies of Mental Health." In *Mind and Body Spaces: Geographies of Illness, Impairment and Disability*, edited by Ruth Butler and Hester Parr, 181–202. Critical Geographies. London: Routledge, 1999.

Parr, Hester, and Chris Philo. *'A Forbidding Fortress of Locks, Bars and Padded Cells': The Locational History of Mental Health Care in Nottingham*. Historical Geography Research Series 32. London: Historical Geography Research Series, 1996.

———. "Mapping 'Mad' Identities." In *Mapping the Subject: Geographies of Cultural Transformation*, edited by Steven Pile and Nigel Thrift, 199–225. London: Routledge, 1995.

Parrott, Fiona. "Mais où a-t-on donc rangé ces souvenirs?" *Ethnologie Française* 37, no. 2 (2007): 305–312.

Parrott, Fiona R. "'It's Not Forever': The Material Culture of Hope." *Journal of Material Culture* 10, no. 3 (2005): 245–262.

———. "'Real Relationships': Sociable Interaction, Material Culture and Imprisonment in a Secure Psychiatric Unit." *Culture, Medicine & Psychiatry* 34 (2010): 555–570.

Patients at Wolston Park Hospital. *In Dark Hours*. Brisbane: Wolston Park Hospital, 1997.

Payne, Christopher. "The State Mental Hospitals: Their Origin, Construction, and Demise." In Payne, *Asylum: Inside*, 7–13.

Payne, Christopher, ed. *Asylum: Inside the Closed World of State Mental Hospitals*. Cambridge, MA: MIT Press, 2009.

Pearce, Susan. "Collecting as Medium and Message." In Hooper-Greenhill, 14–22.

Pearce, Susan M. *Collecting in Contemporary Practice*. London: Sage, 1998.

Pearce, Susan M. *On Collecting. An Investigation into Collecting in the European Tradition*. Collecting Cultures. London and New York: Routledge, 1995.

———. "The Urge to Collect." In *Interpreting Objects and Collections*, ed. Susan M. Pearce, 157–159. Leicester Readers in Museum Studies. London: Routledge, 1994.

Pearce, Susan M., ed. *Experiencing Material Culture in the Western World*. Contemporary Issues in Museum Culture. London: Leicester University Press, 1997.

Pearce, Susan M., and Paul Martin, eds. *The Collector's Voice: Critical Readings in the Practice of Collecting*. Vol. 4: Contemporary Voices. Perspectives on Collecting. Aldershot: Ashgate, 2002.

Peiffer, J. "Assessing Neuropathological Research Carried Out on Victims of the 'Euthanasia' Programme." *Medizinhistorisches Journal* 34 (1999): 339–356.

Penney, Darby, and Peter Stastny. *The Lives They Left Behind: Suitcases From a State Hospital Attic*. New York: Bellevue Literary Press, 2008.

Pink, Sarah. *Home Truths: Gender, Domestic Objects and Everyday Life*. Oxford: Berg, 2004.

Prebble, Kate. "Ordinary Men and Uncommon Women: A History of Psychiatric Nursing in New Zealand Public Mental Hospitals, 1939–1972." Unpublished PhD Thesis, University of Auckland, 1997.

Preuss, Dirk. "Body Worlds: Looking Back and Looking Ahead." *Annals of Anatomy* 190, no. 1 (2008): 23–32.
Pross, Christian. "Nazi Doctors, German Medicine, and Historical Truth." In *The Nazi Doctors and the Nuremberg Code: Human Rights in Human Experimentation*, edited by George J. Annas and Michael A. Grodin. Oxford: Oxford University Press, 1992.
Quirk, Alan, Paul Lelliott, and Clive Seale. "Risk Management by Patients on Psychiatric Wards in London: An Ethnographic Study." *Health, Risk & Society* 7, no. 1 (2005): 85–91.
Radley, Alan. *Works of Illness: Narrative, Picturing and the Social Response to Serious Disease*. Ashby-de-la-Zouch: InkerMen Press, 2009.
Reaume, Geoffrey. "Patients at Work: Insane Asylum Inmates' Labour in Ontario, 1841–1900." In Moran and Wright, 69–96.
———. *Remembrance of Patients Past: Patient Life at the Toronto Hospital for the Insane, 1870–1940*. Canadian Social History. Don Mills: Oxford University Press, 2000.
Redies, Christopher, Michael Viebig, Susanne Zimmermann, and Rosemarie Fröber. "Origin of Corpses Received by the Anatomical Institute at the University of Jena during the Nazi Regime." *Anatomical Record Part B: The New Anatomist* 285B, no. 1 (2005): 6–10.
Reinarz, Jonathan . "The Age of Museum Medicine: The Rise and Fall of the Medical Museum at Birmingham's School of Medicine." *Social History of Medicine* 18, no. 3 (2005): 419–437.
Richardson, Ruth. *Death, Dissection and the Destitute*. Harmondsworth: Penguin, 1987.
———. *Death, Dissection and the Destitute*. 2nd ed. London: Phoenix Press, 2001.
Riegel, Henrietta. "Into the Heart of Irony: Ethnographic Exhibitions and the Politics of Difference." In *Theorizing Museums: Representing Identity and Diversity in a Changing World*, edited by Sharon Macdonald and Gordon Fyfe, 83–104. *Sociological Review* Monographs. Oxford: Blackwell, 1996.
Robertson, George. "Hospital Ideals in the Cure of the Insane: A Statement of Certain Methods in Use at the Stirling District Asylum, Larbert." *Journal of Mental Science* 48 (1902): 261–289.
Robson, Belinda. "Preserving Psychiatry Through Art: Historical Perspectives on the Cunningham Dax Collection of Psychiatric Art." In Coleborne and MacKinnon, *'Madness' in Australia*, 195–205.
Rosenzweig, Roy, and David Thelen. *The Presence of the Past: Popular Uses of History in American Life*. New York: Columbia University Press, 1998.
Rosner, Lisa. *The Anatomy Murders: Being the True and Spectacular History of Edinburgh's Notorious Burke and Hare and of the Man of Science Who Abetted Them in the Commission of Their Most Heinous Crimes*. Philadelphia: University of Pennsylvania Press, 2009.
Rothman, David J. *The Discovery of the Asylum: Social Order and Disorder in the New Republic*. Boston: Little Brown, 1971.
Rubinstein, W. D., and Hilary L. Rubinstein. *Menders of the Mind: A History of the Royal Australian and New Zealand College of Psychiatrists, 1946–1996*. Melbourne: Oxford University Press, 1996.
Sachs, Oliver. "Asylum." In Payne, *Asylum: Inside*, 1–5.
Sandell, Richard, Annie Delin, Jocelyn Dodd, and Jackie Gay. "Beggars, Freaks and Heroes? Museum Collections and the Hidden History of Disability." *Museum Management and Curatorship* 20, no. 1 (2005): 5–19.
Sankey, Ira D., comp. *Sacred Songs and Solos: Revised and Enlarged with Standard Hymns 1200 Pieces*. London: Morgan and Scott, n.d.

Sarat, Austin, Nadav Davidovitch, and Michal Alberstein, eds. *Trauma and Memory: Reading, Healing, and Making Law.* Stanford: Stanford University Press, 2007.

Schlereth, Thomas J. *Cultural History and Material Culture: Everyday Life, Landscapes, Museums.* American Material Culture and Folklife. Charlottesville: University Press of Virginia, 1990.

Scull, Andrew. *Museums of Madness: The Social Organization of Insanity in Nineteenth-Century England.* London: Allen Lane, 1979.

Shevell, Michael I., and Jüergen Peiffer. "Julius Hallervorden's Wartime Activities: Implications for Science Under Dictatorship." *Pediatric Neurology* 25 (2001): 162–165.

Shorter, Edward, ed. *TPH: History and Memories of the Toronto Psychiatric Hospital, 1925–1966.* Toronto: Wall & Emerson, 1996.

Simpson, Moira. *Making Representations: Museums in the Post-Colonial Era.* London: Routledge, 1996.

Snowden, Peter. "Regional Secure Units and Forensic Services in England and Wales." In *Principles and Practice of Forensic Psychiatry*, edited by Robert Bluglass and Paul Bowden, 1375–1387. Edinburgh: Churchill Livingstone, 1990.

Sontag, Susan. *On Photography.* Harmondsworth: Penguin, 1979.

———. *On Photography.* London: Penguin, 2002.

Stanton, Alfred H. and Morris S. Schwartz. *The Mental Hospital: A Study of Psychiatric Participation in Psychiatric illness and Treatment.* New York: Basic Books, 1954.

Stewart, Susan. *On Longing: Narratives of the Miniature, the Gigantic, the Souvenir, the Collection.* Durham: Duke University Press, 1993.

Stoller, Alan. *Report on Mental Health Facilities and Needs of Australia.* Canberra: Printed for the Government of the Commonwealth by A. J. Arthur at the GPO, 1955.

Sturken, Marita. *Tangled Memories: The Vietnam War, the AIDS Epidemic, and the Politics of Remembering.* Berkeley: University of California Press, 1997.

Tacchi, Jo. "Radio Texture: Between Self and Others." In *Material Cultures: Why Some Things Matter*, edited by Daniel Miller, 25–46. London: UCL Press, 1998.

Tagg, John. *The Disciplinary Frame: Photographic Truths and the Capture of Meaning.* Minneapolis: University of Minnesota Press, 2009.

Taylor, Charles. *Modern Social Imaginaries.* Durham: Duke University Press, 2004.

Tomes, Nancy. "The Asylum as Therapeutic Landscape." In Johnson, *Angels in the Architecture*, 1–18.

Trentmann, Frank. "Materiality in the Future of History: Things, Practices, and Politics." *Journal of British Studies* 48, no. 2 (2009): 283–307.

Truscott, M. "Repatriation of Indigenous Cultural Property." Paper prepared for the 2006 Australian State of the Environment Committee, Department of Environment and Heritage, Canberra. http://www.environment.gov.au/soe/2006/publications/emerging/repatriation/index.html (accessed November 18, 2010).

Urry, John. "Gazing on History." In *Representing the Nation: A Reader: Histories, Heritage and Museums.* Edited by David Boswell and Jessica Evans, 208–232. London: Routledge, 1990.

Uzzell, David, and Roy Ballantyne. *Contemporary Issues in Heritage and Environmental Interpretation: Problems and Prospects.* London: Stationery Office, 1998.

Verry, Emma. "The Exposure of Truth: The Use of Photography in Mental Health in the Late Nineteenth and Early Twentieth Century." BA Hons. Diss., University of Otago, 2009.

Viner, Brian. "Television: Our Friends off the North Circular." *The Independent*, March 14, 1999.

Vogel, Susan. "Always True to the Object, in Our Fashion." In Karp and Lavine, 191–204.

Waltenbacher, Thomas. *Zentrale Hinrichtungsstätten. Der Vollzug der Todesstrafe in Deutschland von 1937–1945. Scharfrichter im Dritten Reich*. Berlin: Zwilling, 2008.

Westmore, Ann. "Reading Psychiatry's Archive: Academic Medicine and Psychiatric Medicine in Mid-Twentieth-Century Victoria." In Coleborne and MacKinnon, *‚Madness' in Australia*, 207–216.

Williams, D. J. „The History of Eduard Pernkopf's Topographische Anatomie des Menschen." *Journal of Biocommunication* 15, no. 2 (1988): 2–12.

Williams, Wendy Hunter. *Out of Mind, Out of Sight: The Story of Porirua Hospital*. Porirua: The Hospital, 1987.

Willis, Elizabeth. "Home But Away: Material Evidence of Lives in Victorian Asylums, 1850–1950." *Psychiatry, Psychology and Law* 2, no. 2 (1995): 111–116.

Willis, Elizabeth, and Karen Twigg, eds. *Behind Closed Doors: A Catalogue of Artefacts from Victorian Psychiatric Institutions held at Museum Victoria*. Melbourne: Museum Victoria, 1994.

Wilson, Michael. "'Bodies' Exhibitors Admit Corpse Origins Are Murky." *New York Times*, May 30, 2008. http://www.nytimes.com/ 2008/05/30/nyregion/30bodies.html (accessed June 3, 2008).

Wise, Sarah. *The Italian Boy: Murder and Grave-Robbery in 1830s London*. London: Jonathan Cape, 2004.

Wrigley, June. *The Less Travelled Way*. Melbourne: Collins Dove, 1990.

Wu, Hongda Harry. *Laogai—The Chinese Gulag*. Boulder: Westview Press, 1992.

———. "Using Organs from Executed Prisoners is Unethical." In *Biomedical Ethics: Opposing Viewpoints*, edited by Tamara L. Roleff. San Diego: Greenhaven Press, 1998, 103–107.

Index